Praise for *Fat for Fuel*

"Dr. Joseph Mercola has been a shining beacon of health wisdom and freedom for decades. His latest book, Fat for Fuel, is a masterpiece of cutting-edge research and practical application. This information, if applied, holds the key to sustainable weight loss and enhanced energy. More than that, this lifestyle plan can help reverse chronic illness such as heart disease, diabetes, and even cancer."

— **Christiane Northrup, M.D.**, *New York Times* best-selling author of *Women's Bodies, Women's Wisdom* and *Goddesses Never Age*

"I truly believe that the concept of Mitochondrial Metabolic Therapy will have significant impact on health. As I mentioned in my book, cancer is not likely to occur in people with healthy mitochondria. Dr. Mercola has expanded this concept to a broad range of chronic diseases that involve mitochondrial dysfunction. He provides a clear rationale as well as guidelines for implementation of MMT. This book should be read by anyone interested in maintaining their health without toxic pharmaceuticals."

— **Thomas Seyfried, Ph.D.**, author of *Cancer as a Metabolic Disease* and professor of biology at Boston College

"This remarkable book presents a truly revolutionary program that can help millions of people achieve optimal health. Dr. Mercola clearly explains the importance of mitochondria for metabolic function and carefully guides his readers with detailed practical advice for enhancing their activity. Fat for Fuel *will change the way you think about nutrition and your health."*

— **Leo Galland, M.D.**, author of *The Allergy Solution*

"Dr. Mercola's Fat for Fuel *eloquently presents the leading edge of science, exploring how best to power your body. This is a life-changing text that not only provides a deep dive into why choosing fat as our primary fuel source powerfully correlates with health and disease resistance, but also delivers in terms of how the reader can easily bring about this fundamentally important change. Health, on a global scale, has suffered profoundly as a consequence of commercially influenced dietary recommendations. Mercola's science-based refutation of this status quo provides a welcome and compassionate response, allowing readers to regain and maintain optimal health."*

— **David Perlmutter, M.D., F.A.C.N.**, board-certified neurologist and author of the #1 *New York Times* bestseller *Grain Brain* and *The Grain Brain Whole Life Plan*

"In Fat for Fuel, *Dr. Mercola beautifully lays out the history—and the myths—behind the high-carbohydrate, low-fat diet that has been at the root of so much illness and death in the last half-century. Dr. Mercola is one of the few who have properly understood and embraced my long-standing belief that one's health and lifespan is mostly determined by the proportion of fat versus sugar one burns over a lifetime. He also understands that excess protein creates another whole set of health-eroding issues. Anyone who values their health should read this book."*

— **Ron Rosedale, M.D.**

"Science has already shown that eating fat can make you thin. In this pathbreaking book, Dr. Joseph Mercola goes a critical step further, revealing that using fat as your main fuel source can heal your body at a mitochondrial level, restoring energy and well-being and even helping fight cancer and other diseases. Impeccably researched and passionately argued, Fat for Fuel *dispels dangerous myths about 'healthful' diets, reveals truths the food industry won't tell you about the food you eat, and starts you on a path to radically transforming your health."*

— **Mark Hyman, M.D.**, #1 *New York Times* best-selling author of *Eat Fat Get Thin* and Director of the Cleveland Clinic's Center for Functional Medicine

"The world of nutrition is more confusing than ever. But one thing has become increasingly evident over the past decade: teaching our bodies to use fat instead of glucose as the main fuel source has immense potential to support patients suffering from some of the most devastating chronic diseases. Dr. Mercola's Fat for Fuel *will be an invaluable resource for me in two ways: personally, because I'm a cancer patient myself striving to create an environment that will keep my disease at bay, but also professionally as a nutritional therapist.* Fat for Fuel *will help me inform, educate, and guide my clients."*

— **Patricia Daly, dipNT, mNTOI, mBANT**

"Fat for Fuel *is another fact-based, insightful book by the visionary Joseph Mercola that will not just change your life, but could literally save it. Dr. Mercola understands how food can preserve wellness or destroy it. Boldly challenging old myths about fat, diet, and healing, he gives practical, step-by-step instructions that will empower you to take control of your health whether you are sick and want to get well, or are healthy and want to stay well."*

— **Barbara Loe Fisher**, co-founder, National Vaccine Information Center

"Dr. Mercola's lifetime of research reaches a crescendo with Fat for Fuel. *Every page is a distillation of his genuine passion to optimize human health through diet."*

— **Travis Christofferson**, author of *Tripping over the Truth: How the Metabolic Theory of Cancer Is Overturning One of Medicine's Most Entrenched Paradigms*

"Fat for Fuel is a powerhouse of practical, evidence-based information for the clinician and consumer alike. With so much conflicting information in the nutrition world, this book serves as a critical resource for every physician in training or in practice, and for every person eager to avoid the need for those doctors."

— **Zach Bush, M.D.**, endocrinologist

"Fat for Fuel is a powerful manifesto reexamining the fat-phobic paradigm that has long dominated the thinking about health and nutrition. This is an extremely valuable guidebook for those seeking to understand and implement transformational dietary changes to boost their metabolic and cellular function. By shifting away from the idea of glucose as the optimal source of energy, Dr. Mercola shows how we can harness the benefits of fat and ketones for clean-burning fuel in the quest for optimal health."

— **Michael Stroka, J.D., M.B.A., M.S., C.N.S., L.D.N.**, executive director, Board for Certification of Nutrition Specialists

"In 2017, we have many chronic illness epidemics in the USA. At the center of most of those epidemics is the toxic, nutrient-depleted, dysfunctional human cell. And research is now showing us that the most important organelle in that cell contributing to most of these diseases is the mitochondria. In his book Fat for Fuel, *Joe Mercola has given us a practical blueprint for how to revive our mitochondria using diet as a powerful foundation, with a few other added simple tools, such as intermittent fasting, exercise, light therapy, and some supplemental nutrients. Dr. Mercola tested the Mitochondrial Metabolic Therapy recommendations he makes in this book on himself, with many months of trials and errors and continuous glucose monitoring. He also amassed impressive scientific research from the literature to prove what he recommends on these pages. I highly endorse* Fat for Fuel *as the most practical do-it-yourself guide available today for people to take back control of their health and resolve chronic illnesses."*

— **W. Lee Cowden, M.D., M.D.(H)**, chairman of scientific advisory board, Academy of Comprehensive Integrative Medicine

"Fat for Fuel *is a landmark contribution from Dr. Joe Mercola. . . . Metabolism at its core consists of how our mitochondria utilize nutrients, and Dr. Mercola educates his readers on how to choose the nutrients that optimize mitochondrial function. This book will contribute greatly toward our health goals for our entire population as more and more health-care professionals wake up to this understanding of the importance of optimizing mitochondrial metabolism.* Fat for Fuel *brings mitochondrial function into the mainstream for the healthy benefit of everyone. Bravo!"*

— **J. William (Will) LaValley, M.D.**

"Dr. Mercola proves once again that he is at the very forefront of natural healing and wellness. With medical science understanding more and more how mitochondrial dysfunction leads to chronic disease, Dr. Mercola provides a simple, natural healing plan with this important new book."

— **Jason Fung**, M.D., nephrologist and author of
The Complete Guide to Fasting

"A revolution is growing in medicine, one that revolves around a change from seeing the cell as a membrane-bound bag of water controlled by the all-powerful DNA to a more fluid conception of the cell centered on the central role of the mitochondria. Dr. Mercola is at the forefront of this exciting revolution, and this book gives you both the theoretical basis and practical suggestions for supporting your mitochondria and regaining better health. I would encourage everyone to read this book and strongly consider following Dr. Mercola's many helpful suggestions and guidelines."

— **Thomas Cowan, M.D.**

"A book like Fat for Fuel *has been a long time coming. Backed by a wealth of research, Dr. Mercola makes the definitive case that fat, not sugar, is the power source on which our bodies are meant to run, and he outlines what changes we can make in our daily lives to use fat as fuel. KU Integrative Medicine has been waiting for this book!"*

— **Jeanne A. Drisko**, M.D., C.N.S, F.A.C.N., Director, KU Integrative Medicine, and Riordan endowed professor of orthomolecular medicine, University of Kansas Medical Center

"Dr. Mercola is one of the most brilliant minds in modern medicine, and he has achieved a true masterpiece with Fat for Fuel. Why? The book defies the status quo and reveals the truth behind everything from why fasting is a healthy habit to why you need to become a fat-burning machine. He even shocks us with the details on how iron can negatively impact mitochondrial health (you'll be surprised). This book is a must-read if you want to optimize your body and brain while systematically eliminating a host of risk factors for chronic disease."

— **Ben Greenfield**, BenGreenfieldFitness.com (Dr. Mercola's favorite fitness podcast)

"Fat for Fuel is a crucial read to obtain and maintain health, especially in the modern pandemic of inflammation-driven chronic diseases. This important book teaches principles most people have not yet heard and extends its reach beyond the small group of practitioners around the world who are already utilizing these methods. Implementing the principles outlined in this book has proved life-changing for thousands and I now expect that this information will transform millions. These tools and strategies are 'the real deal,' and a proven answer to our current state of dis-ease. The science presented here is clear and well-documented and will change the way you think about what really brings you health and healing."

— **Daniel Pompa**, D.C.

"Fat for Fuel comes at the perfect time. With the cost of health care soaring, we have to take responsibility for protecting our health instead of simply treating disease. Understanding the mechanisms of how we function is essential to a healthy body and brain, and modern-day revolutionary Dr. Mercola has relentlessly dug through the research to bring this latest and greatest knowledge of our bodies to the bookshelf. Not only does this page-turner highlight the need for fat in our diet, it shows us how to prepare our bodies to process and utilize it most efficiently—a key ingredient in the overall strategy to attain optimal health."

— **Erin Elizabeth**, investigative journalist, author of In the Lymelight, and founder of HealthNutNews.com

FAT
FOR
FUEL

ALSO BY DR. JOSEPH MERCOLA

Effortless Healing

The No-Grain Diet

Take Control of Your Health

Sweet Deception

Dark Deception

The Great Bird Flu Hoax

Freedom at Your Fingertips

Generation XL

Healthy Recipes for Your Nutritional Type

♦ ♦

FAT

FOR

FUEL

A Revolutionary Diet to Combat
Cancer, Boost Brain Power,
and Increase Your Energy

DR. JOSEPH MERCOLA

HAY HOUSE, INC.
Carlsbad, California • New York City
London • Sydney • New Delhi

Library of Congress has cataloged the earlier edition as follows:

Names: Mercola, Joseph.
Title: Fat for fuel : a revolutionary diet to combat cancer, boost brain
   power, and increase your energy / Joseph Mercola.
Description: Carlsbad, California : Hay House, Inc., 2017.
Identifiers: LCCN 2016057555 | ISBN 9781401953775 (hardback)
Subjects: LCSH: Diet therapy. | Mitochondrial pathology. | Metabolism. |
   BISAC: HEALTH & FITNESS / Alternative Therapies. | MEDICAL / Endocrinology
   & Metabolism. | HEALTH & FITNESS / Diets.
Classification: LCC RM214 .M47 2017 | DDC 613.2/5--dc23 LC record available at
   https://lccn.loc.gov/2016057555

Tradepaper ISBN: 978-1-4019-5424-6
E-book ISBN: 978-1-4019-5378-2
Audiobook ISBN: 978-1-4019-5379-9

10 9 8 7 6 5 4 3 2 1
1st edition, May 2017
2nd edition, December 2018

Printed in the United States of America

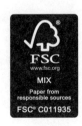 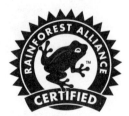

This book is dedicated to all of our friends, family, and loved ones we've lost bravely battling cancer.

CONTENTS

INTRODUCTION

I have been passionate about learning about health for the last 50 years. I hope my story will prevent you from making some of the same painful and foolish mistakes I have made along my journey toward optimal health. It is my experience that it is far easier and less painful to learn from others' mistakes.

My commitment to a fitness routine started in 1968. Dr. Ken Cooper's book *Aerobics* catalyzed my interest in health, which eventually led me to enter medical school 10 years later. Sadly, like most health enthusiasts during the late '60s and early '70s, I fell in line with the low-fat, high-carb diet that has been popularized by the mass media for decades. This type of diet is the polar opposite of what I now understand as necessary to prevent chronic disease, manage cancer, and optimize health.

Seven years of medical school and family practice residency solidified my brainwashing into the conventional drug-based medical model that exists primarily to treat the symptoms of disease. Virtually none of my seven years of training ever addressed the root cause of common chronic illness. Rather, it focused on managing symptoms through the use of pharmaceutical products and medical procedures.

In 1995, my understanding made a radical leap in evolution. I met Dr. Ron Rosedale in a room with a few dozen other physicians at a meeting of the Great Lakes Academy of Medicine. Little did I realize then how fortunate I was to be one of the first physicians inspired by Dr. Rosedale's wisdom on clinical metabolic biochemistry.

Dr. Rosedale lectured for over three hours on the critical need to control high insulin levels in order to prevent nearly every chronic degenerative disease that is rampant in our modern culture, including diabetes, obesity, heart disease, cancer, arthritis, and neurodegenerative diseases.

You may have had a similar epiphany in your life when you knew you were encountering a foundational truth. In this case I knew it could impact the health of hundreds of millions of people who desperately needed help.

For the next ten years I used the principles Dr. Rosedale taught me along with other information I had gained from attending many dozens of postgraduate courses on nutrition—a subject, suffice to say, never taught in medical school—to continually refine my understanding and use of food as medicine. (Even today most medical schools fail to provide even the most rudimentary basics of nutrition.[1])

I was fortunate to have the privilege of using these principles to care for more than 25,000 patients in my clinical career. It was enormously rewarding to be able to provide solutions for most of my patients, many of whom had been seen but not successfully treated by some of the leading physicians at some of the finest institutions in the country.

It wasn't that I was any smarter than these other physicians—far from it. The difference was that I stayed disciplined, open-minded, and diligent in pursuing the truth about the underpinnings of health. My unfair advantage was elemental: I had a better understanding of how the body healed itself because I had made a decision to stay at arm's length from pharmaceutical interests. That perspective helped me focus on looking for and remedying the cause of disease rather than mitigating the symptoms.

Although I was aware of the importance of limiting refined carbs and processed foods and replacing them with healthier choices, I was relatively clueless about the importance of eating plenty of high-quality fats and activating the body's natural ability to burn fat for its primary fuel instead of glucose. I didn't realize that I still had to look further.

WE'RE LOSING THE WAR ON CANCER BECAUSE WE'VE BEEN FIGHTING THE WRONG ENEMY

Twenty years after I learned of the importance of insulin, I read Travis Christofferson's *Tripping over the Truth: How the Metabolic Theory of Cancer Is Overturning One of Medicine's Most Entrenched Paradigms*. I was struck by an epiphany similar to when I first heard Dr. Rosedale's lecture—here was something that had the potential to radically improve the health of millions.

The argument Christofferson so eloquently laid out—and that builds on what Dr. Rosedale taught me in 1995—is that cancer and nearly all other chronic diseases are caused by defective metabolic processes in your mitochondria. This is typically a result of insulin and leptin receptor resistance from too many net carbs and activation of the mTOR metabolic signaling pathway by excessive protein. We will go into great detail on these topics later on, but for now it's enough to know that this is the root of the problem for most.

This is in direct opposition to the conventional views of the roots of disease; for over a century, the widely accepted scientific dogma has been that cancer is a genetic disease that develops as a result of chromosomal damage in the nucleus of the cell. The discovery of the structure of DNA by Watson and Crick in the mid-20th century along with DNA sequencing in the 21st century has served to greatly reinforce this viewpoint.

Tragically, President Nixon's War on Cancer, which started with the signing of the National Cancer Act in 1971, has been a miserable failure. And in 2016, President Obama's moonshot to cure cancer is doomed to this same fate, despite its billion-dollar price tag. Today, in the United States alone, over 1,600 people will die from cancer.[2] If you look at global statistics, that number jumps to an astonishing 21,000 who pass each day from this mostly preventable disease.[3] The odds are astronomically high that at some point in your life you will develop cancer or know someone who has cancer. Shockingly, the latest data from 2011 to 2013 show that nearly 40 percent of us will be diagnosed with cancer at some point during our lifetime.[4] I have come to see that we are losing the war against cancer because scientists are chasing a flawed paradigm: most adult cancers are not a disease of damaged DNA, but rather one of defective metabolism.

THE MIGHTY MITOCHONDRIA

Mitochondria—tiny energy factories within your cells that use a metabolic process to convert the food you eat and the air you breathe into energy—are at the core of what is causing your biological systems to go haywire in the first place, making you vulnerable to cancer and most other chronic diseases. When large numbers of mitochondria in your body stop functioning properly, it is simply impossible to stay healthy. This is an enormously empowering shift in how we approach cancer and all chronic diseases: if disease starts as a result of metabolic dysfunction, we can heal that dysfunction. How? That's what this book will show you—how to carefully choose nutrients and employ other strategies that turn on your body's innate ability to prevent and heal from disease.

In its most distilled form, the theory that drives this book is that the food choices you make every day directly impact your mitochondria. And if you make food choices that boost the health of your mitochondria, you also make it much less likely that the genetic material that's housed in your mitochondria will become damaged and trigger a chain reaction that is more likely than not to result in disease.

Another major impetus for me to write this book was seeing so many friends and colleagues, including Jerry Burnetti, die from cancer. It is no exaggeration to say that Jerry was a genius. He was one of the world's leading experts on regenerative farming, and I had the privilege of interviewing him for my website a few years ago.

Seeing the movie *The Fault in Our Stars*, a devastating romantic tragedy about two teens with cancer who find each other and fall in love despite their imminent mortality, was another catalyst for me. Though incredibly sad, it is one of my favorite movies. If you haven't already seen it or read the book, I strongly encourage you to do so.

I believe—as do many of the experts I interviewed for this book—that tragic scenarios like Jerry's early death and the story depicted in this tearjerker film are unnecessary because more than 90 percent of cancer cases are either preventable or treatable. I had to do something to help staunch the loss of so many talented and loving people to cancer.

Since viewing the movie and reading Travis's book, I have scoured the National Library of Medicine for the latest research, which has led me to hundreds of review articles on the critical role of mitochondria and what factors play into how best to optimize their function. I have gained insights via personal interviews of many of the most respected authorities in this area.

One of these is Miriam Kalamian, Ed.M., M.S., C.N.S., a nutrition consultant, educator, and author specializing in the implementation of ketogenic therapies for people with cancer. Miriam is the go-to nutrition consultant for Dr. Thomas Seyfried, who is widely recognized as one of the leading pioneers in the metabolic theory of cancer. She has worked with hundreds of clients to adopt the food changes I outline in this book, and she has contributed invaluable insight and information that you will read in the pages to come. She played a vital role in helping me use what I've learned to put the puzzle pieces together for you.

THE EATING PROGRAM THAT CAN HEAL YOUR METABOLISM

My goal in writing this book is to present you with a clear, simple, and rational explanation based on science that will help you understand how your body works at a biological and molecular level. I will also tell you what foods to eat, practical strategies to follow, and ways to monitor your progress to help your mitochondria thrive—a program I call Mitochondrial Metabolic Therapy (MMT).

Simply put, MMT is a system of eating that will help shift your metabolism from burning glucose as your primary fuel to burning fat to fuel your body. When you make this shift, you optimize your mitochondrial function and protect your mitochondrial DNA from potential damage that could lead to disease.

At its most basic level, MMT is a high-fat, adequate-protein, low-carb diet that is built on eating the highest-quality foods available. It is quite a shift from the typical American diet—which is notorious for its excessive refined grains, sugars, and low-quality fats. As you will see, the foods that make up MMT are delicious. Luscious, even. They are satisfying, satiating, and absolutely energizing. And once you make the change to MMT, you will finally be free of hunger, cravings, and any feelings of deprivation that accompany the vast majority of eating plans, aka "diets," out there.

MMT is about so much more than the foods you eat—it factors in *when* you eat as well, as regular periods of fasting improve mitochondrial function and accelerate the transition from burning sugar to burning fat. (I cover fasting extensively in Chapter 10, but at this point, you can rest assured that MMT does not require you to go even a whole day without eating; most of your fasting hours are spent sleeping.)

MMT is for you if you are facing one or more serious health conditions—such as cancer, type 2 diabetes, neurodegenerative disease including Alzheimer's and other forms of dementia, or obesity—or you are passionate about optimizing your health while also slowing down the aging process.

MMT, in whole or part, is optional. And options are wonderful things to have. Perhaps you don't fit into either the chronically ill or the passionate-about-health category right now. But should you find yourself at that point later, or desire to prevent a health crisis, you'll know that there is a powerful healing protocol available, one that puts you in control. That is no small thing.

THIS IS EMERGING SCIENCE—
BUT YOU CAN REAP THE BENEFITS NOW

Please understand that mitochondrial and metabolic health is an emerging discipline and only a handful of researchers and even fewer practicing physicians are actively involved in its study. But I firmly believe that at some point in the future, metabolic therapy will be accepted as the standard of care not only for cancer but for most chronic diseases.

Thankfully you and your family don't have to wait 10 or 20 years to reap those benefits. You can begin to improve your health, prevent needless pain and suffering, and help lower your risk of developing serious diseases like cancer by applying what we already know about mitochondrial dysfunction today.

I fully realize that much of the information in this book is not widely accepted yet by the mainstream and many will criticize it. I and others pioneering the way forward toward a more inclusive and holistic view of health and healing are very accustomed to this type of reaction when we provide evidence that there is a more rational and safer way to stay healthy.

The first time I experienced this was as a medical student in the early 1980s when I recommended improving gut microflora as a way to treat ulcers rather than using prescription drugs. I was widely criticized by all of my supervising physicians for promoting this new idea. Years later, I was vindicated when it eventually became the standard of care. Dr. Barry Marshall was the courageous family physician who had pointed me in this direction, and 25 years later in 2005, he won the Nobel Prize in Medicine.

Similarly, I was the first to publicly warn of the dangers of the anti-inflammatory drug Vioxx. One year before the drug was approved for sale in the U.S., I told my newsletter readers that this was a dangerous drug that could cause heart disease and stroke. Sure enough, four years after Vioxx was released Merck voluntarily withdrew it from the market—but not before it killed an estimated 60,000 people.[5]

There are many examples in the history of medicine where routine use of pharmaceutical products and other medical interventions is accepted as "standard of care" for a period of time before they are found to be flat-out wrong and toxic to human health.

I believe it is time to challenge widely accepted assumptions about the causes and cures for cancer. We must open our minds and reexamine the evidence by first acknowledging that science is never settled and that our current understanding of biology is rapidly evolving as more objective, impartial, and unbiased research is performed and published.

I was initially reluctant to write a book about mitochondria dysfunction and cancer because of the very real potential for the information to rapidly become outdated. I thought it was far more efficient and effective to give away the information in real time on the Internet on my website, which I started in 1997 in my off hours as a medical practitioner and which has grown into one of the most visited health sites in the world, with over 15 million unique visitors and 40 million page views a month. But my team convinced me about 10 years ago that books serve a very valuable purpose. They require the author to consolidate thoughts into a comprehensive printed resource where all the material is carefully integrated into an easy-to-follow format.

I am still concerned that the information in this book will need to be revised in the not too distant future, but it will likely be several years before I can carve out the time to fully update it. That is why I strongly encourage you to stay on top of the emerging science by subscribing to my free newsletter or doing your own searches at mercola.com, and, of course, reading from many other sources to help educate and empower yourself and your family on health care and health-related issues.

I continue to network with the leading researchers studying metabolic disease, and I actively review new studies as they are published. I will regularly post updates in my free newsletter at mercola.com, so you will be one of the first to know about new scientific developments and revised recommendations. It has been so rewarding to see what an impact this information has already had in helping people gain awareness, empower themselves, and recapture their health without the use of potentially toxic and dangerous pharmaceutical products. I hope that this book will help millions more do the same.

PART I

RESCUING YOUR METABOLISM

CHAPTER 1

THE TRUTH ABOUT MITOCHONDRIA, FREE RADICALS, AND DIETARY FATS

Because you are reading this book, I am assuming two things about you:

- You recognize the link between the food you eat and your health.
- You have faced at least one health crisis, either your own or that of someone you love.

I'm also fairly certain that you are confused about what to eat in order to regain your health. I get it. Honestly, I don't see how you could avoid feeling at a loss here, as the food and pharmaceutical industries have effectively manipulated the conversation—and lobbied the government—to distort the truth in the quest to benefit their bottom line.

They have systematically and intentionally misled you about what is healthy and what isn't.

I spend the majority of my free waking hours reading the research and interviewing leading scientists in these areas. Even though I am trained as a family physician and have treated over 25,000 patients, I am still continuously refining and rethinking my understanding of what a healthy diet truly is.

In this chapter, I'm going to explain a few key concepts to arm you with the reasons *why* the eating plan I'll outline in the second half of this book works to restore health and ward off disease. First, I'll cover exactly what mitochondria are, and then I'll explain how fat can be either a friend or a foe depending on what type of fat it is and how it is processed—and how the nutritional guidance we've received from medical associations, doctors, mainstream media, and the government have led us astray. By the end of this chapter, I hope you'll have a clear understanding of why it's so important to take care of your mitochondria, and exactly how harmful a typical American diet is to these tiny physiological wonders.

Meet Your Mitochondria

Perhaps you recall hearing about mitochondria in your high school biology class or have read about mitochondrial disease on the Internet, but you are still not quite sure what mitochondria are or what function they serve. Mitochondria are so vital to your health that if you are interested in warding off and healing from disease, it is critical for you to learn more about them.

Mitochondria are tiny organelles (think of them as micro-organs) contained within nearly all your cells. One of their many critical roles is to produce energy by combining nutrients from the sugars and fats you eat with oxygen from the air you breathe.

Researchers estimate that mitochondria account for 10 percent of your body weight, with approximately 10 million billion within the cells of an average adult.[1] If that number is hard to comprehend, consider that more than 1 billion mitochondria would fit on the head of a pin.

Some cells have more mitochondria than others. For example, female germ cells, known as oocytes, have hundreds of thousands, while mature red blood cells and skin cells have few to none. Most cells, including liver cells, have somewhere between 80 and 2,000 mitochondria. The more metabolically active cells are—such as those found in the heart, brain, liver, kidneys, and muscles—the more mitochondria they have. You can imagine, then, that having healthy, well-functioning mitochondria will have a wide-ranging and powerfully positive impact on your overall health.

Mitochondria continuously generate energy molecules called adenosine triphosphate (ATP). Are you curious, as I was, to know how much ATP is actually generated? I suspect you will be surprised to learn that your mitochondria produce about 110 pounds of ATP *every day*.[2]

According to *Power, Sex, Suicide*, Nick Lane's excellent book on mitochondria, this enormous army of organelles is hard at work every second of the day, pumping out 10,000 times more energy, gram for gram, than the sun. Every second!

So you can appreciate that optimal mitochondrial function is key to a well-functioning metabolism. Repairing mitochondrial dysfunction offers one of the simplest and most promising new strategies for improving your health and helping prevent diseases like cancer from developing in your body in the first place.

THE IMPORTANT ROLE OF FREE RADICALS IN MITOCHONDRIAL ENERGY PRODUCTION

Every cell in your body needs a continuous supply of energy. Most of that energy is produced by your mitochondria through a process that involves two essential biological functions required to sustain life: breathing and eating. This process is called oxidative phosphorylation, and it is responsible for producing energy in the form of ATP.

(This process is in contrast to cancer cells, which rely more on metabolizing glucose outside of the mitochondria to produce energy in a less efficient process called glycolysis.)

ATP, the "the currency of energy," drives essentially every biological process in your body, from the function of your brain to the beating of your heart. Your heart has more than 5,000 mitochondria per cell, for example, making it the most energy-dense tissue in your body.

During oxidative phosphorylation, your mitochondria host a complex series of chemical reactions, which can be challenging to understand even for most biochemistry students, called the Krebs cycle and the electron transport chain. Combined, these reactions use electrons liberated from the food you eat and protons contained within the cycle to produce energy and keep the process rolling. At the end of the chain, electrons react with oxygen to form water.

A percentage of electrons will leak from the electron transport chain and form what is called reactive oxygen species (ROS). ROS are molecules that contain oxygen atoms that have gained one or more unpaired electrons, making them very unstable. These highly reactive atoms form potentially destructive free radicals. You are likely familiar with the term *free radicals*. You may even believe that they are universally dangerous and supplement with antioxidants to neutralize them. (I will explain why this isn't necessarily so in just a few moments.)

Free radicals react with other molecules in what are known as oxidation reactions in order to neutralize their unstable electrical charge. Oxidation is essentially "biological rusting." It creates a snowball effect—as molecules steal electrons from one another, each one becomes a new free radical, leaving behind a trail of biological carnage. This rapidly expanding horde of free radicals collects within the cell and degrades cell and mitochondrial membranes in a process known as lipid peroxidation. When this happens, the membranes become brittle and leaky, causing them to disintegrate.

Free radicals can also damage your DNA by disrupting replication, interfering with its maintenance activities, and altering its structure. Current research estimates that your DNA suffers a free radical attack somewhere between 10,000 and 100,000 times a day, or nearly *one assault every second*.[3]

All of these factors can lead to tissue degradation, which increases your risk of disease. In fact, free radicals are linked to over 60 different diseases, including:

- Alzheimer's disease
- Atherosclerosis and heart disease
- Cancer
- Cataracts
- Parkinson's disease

As you can imagine, free radicals have an enormous impact on your health, and the startling fact is that approximately 90 percent or more of the ROS in your body are produced within your mitochondria.

But it is also true that free radicals play a role in health and not just disease. Under normal physiological conditions, they actually play many very valuable roles in your body.

- They regulate many crucial cellular functions, such as the creation of melatonin and nitric oxide, and the optimization of important metabolic signaling pathways that regulate functions such as hunger, fat storage, and aging.

- They act as natural biological signals that respond to environmental stressors such as toxins and chemicals in cigarette smoke and the environment.

- They are responsible for the anticancer effects of pro-oxidative chemotherapy drugs.

- They play a role in the beneficial effects of exercise, as your body produces more free radicals when you exercise, simply due to the increase in mitochondrial energy production.

So it's not that ROS are to be avoided at all costs. It's not ROS in general that are harmful; it's ROS *in excess* that are damaging to your health. The point is you can use MMT to optimize the generation and reduction of ROS in your cells. Think of it as the "Goldilocks phenomenon": not too much and not too little but "just right" amounts of ROS being made by your healthy mitochondria.

Thus, if you indiscriminately suppress free radicals, you can actually run into complications with the law of unintended consequences. This is why the popular approach to reducing free radicals by loading your body with antioxidant supplements—which can neutralize too many of these free radicals—can easily backfire when they suppress these other important functions of free radicals.

One example of the adverse consequences of excessive antioxidants would be the neutralization of the desirable ROS in cancer cell mitochondria. When these free radicals build up, they cause cancer cells to self-destruct via apoptosis (automatic programmed cell death).

If you have been diagnosed with cancer, check with your licensed health care practitioner about limiting antioxidants including vitamin C, vitamin E, selenium, and especially N-acetyl-cysteine in order to avoid conferring survival advantage to the cancer cells. However, high dose IV vitamin C or oral liposomal C is used by many integrative cancer physicians to treat cancer as the vitamin C turns to hydrogen peroxide, which kills many cancer cells. If your physician does not yet know this molecular biology, perhaps you can suggest they read this chapter to become familiar with this important biological information.

THE DIETARY KEY TO LIMITING FREE RADICALS WITHOUT SUPPLEMENTS

So how can you keep the proper balance of ROS? Fortunately the answer is quite simple. Rather than suppress excessive free radicals with antioxidants, the ideal solution is to produce fewer of them in the first place.

This is why your food choices are so important: the primary benefit of eating a diet high in quality fats, low in net carbs (total carbs minus fiber), and adequate in protein—such as MMT, the eating plan I outline in the second part of this book—is that it optimizes the capacity of your mitochondria to generate a fuel known as ketones that, in conjunction with low blood glucose levels, produces far fewer ROS and secondary free radicals than when you eat primarily carbohydrates.

In other words, carbs can be seen as a far dirtier fuel than fats. When you adopt a high-fat, low-carb diet and make the switch to burning fat and ketones for fuel instead of glucose, your mitochondria's exposure to oxidative damage drops by as much as 30 to 40 percent compared to when your primary source of fuel is sugar, as is typical in American diets today. This means that when you are "fat adapted"—that is, when you have made the transition to burning fat for fuel—your mitochondrial DNA, cell membranes, and protein can remain stronger, healthier, and more resilient.

In order to regain your body's ability to burn ketones as your primary fuel, you must focus on increasing your intake of healthy fats and decreasing your consumption of carbs in order to keep your blood glucose levels low. This is what Mitochondrial Metabolic Therapy is engineered to do.

The only catch is that when you replace carbs with fat, you must do it with care. The fats you choose must be high quality and, ideally, organic. But most importantly, they should not be industrially processed omega-6 vegetable oils, for reasons that I'll cover in just a moment.

You likely realize that espousing a high-fat diet massively contradicts the conventional nutrition guidelines and public health messages of the last half-century. Thankfully that is changing, albeit slowly. But in order to truly empower you to have the courage and knowledge to buck conventional dietary wisdom, we need to look back at how these guidelines became so prevalent. In the next section I will briefly summarize the health crisis that has occurred over the past 70 years in the United States as a direct result of recommendations to consume a low-fat diet.

Let's start at the beginning of the 20th century.

The American Table in the Early 1900s

In the late 1800s, the majority of Americans were either farmers themselves or lived in rural communities that depended on farmers for their food. There were a few commercially processed foods available: Kellogg's developed corn flakes in 1898,[4] companies such as Heinz, Libby's, and Campbell's had been selling canned foods for decades already, and deodorized cottonseed oil—otherwise known as Wesson Oil—came on the market in 1899.[5] But the majority of foods on American tables were whole, unprocessed, and locally grown. Interestingly, they were also organic as synthetic fertilizers and pesticides had not yet been introduced.

Cottonseed oil, before appearing in American kitchens in the familiar Wesson bottle, was a waste product of the cotton industry that was used primarily in soap and as fuel for lamps. As electricity became more available and affordable during the first decades of the 20th century, manufacturers had a glut of cottonseed oil on their hands—an ample supply in search of demand.

Cottonseed oil in its natural state is cloudy and has a red tint due to the presence of gossypol, a naturally occurring phytochemical that is toxic to animals, so manufacturers had to develop a deodorizing process to make cottonseed oil palatable as a food product.[6] One turn-of-the-century article from *Popular Science* summed up perfectly the process of taking cottonseed oil from waste bin to table: "What was garbage in 1860 was fertilizer in 1870, cattle feed in 1880, and table food and many things else in 1890."[7]

Cottonseed oil wasn't only unpalatable in its natural state. It came with serious issues due to the fact that it, like nearly all vegetable oils, is a polyunsaturated fatty acid (PUFA), meaning that it has multiple (which is what "poly" means) double bonds between atoms in its molecular structure (meaning the atoms are "unsaturated"). These double bonds are vulnerable to attack by free radicals, which then cause damage to the molecule. When you eat too many PUFAs, they are increasingly incorporated into your cell membranes. Because these fats are unstable, your cells become fragile and prone to oxidation, which leads to all sorts of health problems, such as chronic inflammation and atherosclerosis.

This instability means that vegetable oils are also prone to going rancid. This made them less appealing to food manufacturers because the rise of railroads and refrigeration meant that food could be trucked long distances and sit on shelves for weeks. This is why hydrogenated fats were first heralded as a godsend: they eliminated the vulnerable double bonds and made vegetable oils shelf stable.

In 1907, the Cincinnati-based soap company Procter & Gamble was approached by Edwin Kayser, a German chemist who claimed he had developed a process for making liquid fats solid and shelf stable. The company purchased the U.S. rights to the process and began experimenting, at first in search of a way to make cheaper and more appealing-looking soap.[8]

Once hydrogenated cottonseed oil was developed, however, P&G realized it had the same luminous white look as lard, the most popular cooking fat at the time. Why not sell it as a cooking fat? In 1910, P&G applied for a patent for Crisco—hydrogenated cottonseed oil, what we know today as a trans fat—and the shift away from animal fats to industrially processed vegetable fats began in earnest.

When Procter & Gamble debuted Crisco in 1911,[9] they introduced it to the public as "the ideal fat," notable for its "purity" and for being "absolutely all vegetable."[10] As a result of these marketing efforts, sales jumped from 2.6 million pounds in 1912 to 60 million pounds four years later.[11]

Where the average American consumed just under 9 pounds of industrially processed fats—from margarine and vegetable oil—a year in 1909, that number would zoom to about 20 pounds per year by 1950, 15 of them from hydrogenated oils and 5 from vegetable oils.[12] All manner of oils, including those derived from soybeans and corn, were hydrogenated and sold in the form of Crisco, margarine, and a variety of packaged, frozen, and fried foods.

As we began consuming more omega-6 vegetable oils than ever before in human history, three other technological developments further changed the nature of the food we ate: synthetic fertilizers, food additives, and pesticides—primarily Roundup.

- **Synthetic fertilizers** were developed to help farmers produce ever higher yields of ever fewer types of crops. The use of synthetic fertilizers decimated soil microbes and their ability to mineralize the soil, which contributed to profoundly mineral deficient soils that were unable to produce nutrient-dense crops.

  They also made it possible for farmers to focus on growing only one or two crops—such as corn and soy—instead of the traditional method of rotating through a large number of different crops in an effort stave off soil depletion. This is yet another way the growing supply of vegetable oils created a demand for them.

- **Food additives** were added to the food supply at a record clip over the first half of the 20th century. By 1958, nearly 800 food additives were being used with little oversight or concern for safety. Consumer complaints from food- and drug-related symptoms grew to the point that Congress passed the Food Additives Amendment.[13] This legislation required food manufacturers to prove the safety of any food additives before they brought their product to market.

  It also created a loophole: any additive that was "generally regarded as safe" (GRAS) by the scientific community or was in widespread use in food before 1958 could be added to food products without first being approved by, or even disclosed to, the FDA. Still today, with an estimated 10,000 chemicals commonly used in the food supply, there are at least 1,000 that the FDA has never reviewed.[14]

  Even additives that do not make the GRAS list are often exempt from scientific scrutiny, as the FDA allows companies to perform their own studies. One of the most egregious examples of an unsafe additive that the food industry preemptively declared safe is trans fats. We now know trans fats are a prime driver of inflammation and are linked to increases in heart disease,[15] insulin resistance,[16] obesity,[17] and Alzheimer's disease.[18]

It makes you wonder what else is on that list, doesn't it?

- **Glyphosate**—the main active ingredient in the toxic herbicide Roundup—is an enormous threat to your mitochondrial health. Because many vegetable oils, and the processed foods that contain them, are made out of genetically modified corn, soybeans, and canola, they are highly likely to be contaminated with this ubiquitous chemical. This is dire news, given that nearly 2 million tons of glyphosate have been dumped into American soil from 1974 to 2016.[19] Worldwide, nearly 10 million tons have been applied in that same time frame.

There are two main ways glyphosate damages your mitochondria:

- The first involves manganese, a mineral that our bodies need in small amounts for healthy bones, immune function, and neutralization of free radicals.

  Glyphosate binds manganese and many other important minerals in plants sprayed with Roundup, with the result that a creature that eats the plants will not get the benefit of these minerals.

  Glyphosate can also bind to and deplete these minerals from your body. This is a problem because your mitochondria require manganese to convert superoxide, a potentially harmful by-product of oxygen metabolism, into water. This is a critical process that protects your mitochondria from oxidative damage. Without manganese, this mechanism is severely compromised.

- Glyphosate also interferes with ATP production by affecting your mitochondrial membranes. When coupled with the so-called inert solvents included in Roundup, the toxicity of glyphosate is magnified as much as 2,000-fold.[20] This makes the membrane more permeable, allowing the glyphosate to go straight to the heart of the mitochondria.

Saturated Fat Becomes the Enemy

What's interesting is that despite manufacturers' claims that refined vegetable oils were healthful, Americans experienced a massive uptick in heart disease during the first half of the 20th century. And although these oils were a new introduction to the food supply, no one thought to question their role in this new epidemic. Rather, a familiar and previously ubiquitous nutrient took the blame, mostly due to the haphazard and apparently biased research of one man.

Our decades-long mortal fear of fat was born in 1951, when an American physiology professor named Ancel Keys went to Europe in search of the root of heart disease. Keys had heard that Naples, Italy, had a low rate of cardiovascular disease, so he went to observe the eating habits of the Neapolitans.

Remember that Europe had been decimated during World War II—all manner of infrastructure had been destroyed during fighting—and for many years after peace was proclaimed, famine conditions existed. These conditions were the worst and most persistent in Greece and Italy, which had the least amount of food per capita in all of Europe, according to a 1951 survey. These were the finite and unusual circumstances that Keys waltzed into, which he perceived as long-standing tradition that he would eventually codify into "the Mediterranean Diet."

In Naples, Keys noticed that residents dined primarily on pasta and plain pizza, accompanied by vegetables drizzled in olive oil, cheese, fruit for dessert, plenty of wine, and very little meat, "except among the small class of rich people . . . they ate meat every day instead of every week or two," he wrote.

Keys's wife, a medical technologist, conducted an informal study on the Neapolitans' serum levels of cholesterol and "found them to be very low except among members of the Rotary Club"— the class of people who could afford to eat meat. This less-than-rigorous scientific approach led Keys to deduce that avoiding meat resulted in a lower incidence of heart attacks; somehow the prevalence of cheese in the diet (also a source of saturated fat) escaped his notice, but he would soon prove himself skilled at ignoring evidence that didn't confirm his biases.[21]

After Italy, Keys continued looking for proof that a diet high in saturated fat was associated with a high rate of cardiovascular disease, compiling data from six countries with high rates of heart disease and diets typically high in saturated fats.[22] The evidence seemed compelling, logical even. For instance, men in America— who ate a diet high in saturated fat—died from cardiovascular disease at a much higher rate than men in Japan, who ate little saturated fat.

But the evidence was skewed. Keys didn't include other facts, such as that the Japanese also ate far less sugar and processed foods; in fact, they ate far less food in general than their contemporaries. Keys also didn't include countries that didn't fit his mold, such as France, where consumption of saturated fat was high and cardiovascular deaths low. (Instead, this finding was later described as "the French Paradox.") Still, his ideas gained traction as he published numerous papers and best-selling books espousing a link between saturated fats and degenerative heart disease.

Keys was also a master at ingratiating himself to people and positions of power. When President Eisenhower had a massive heart attack in 1955, Keys had the ear of Paul Dudley White, the president's personal physician. At the following day's news conference, White advised the public to eat less saturated fat and cholesterol to prevent heart disease—recommendations he got directly from Keys.[23]

Keys also used his connections and influence to join the nutrition committee of the American Heart Association (AHA), which, based on Keys's input, issued a report in 1961 that counseled patients with a high risk of heart disease to cut down on saturated fat.[24] (It's distressing to note that the AHA began its rise to prominence in 1948, the same year Procter & Gamble donated over $1.7 million to it[25]—making the AHA seriously indebted to the makers of Crisco.)

Nineteen sixty-one was also the year *Time* magazine put Keys on its cover wearing a white lab coat, hailing him as "the twentieth century's most influential nutrition expert."

In 1970, Keys went on to publish the Seven Countries Study,[26] which elaborated on his original research of six countries, and it was a shot heard round the world—it has now been cited in over a million other studies. Even though Keys's scientific research never proved causation, only association, between saturated fat and heart disease, he won the battle of public opinion. And we are still paying the price.

Thanks in large part to Keys, the American medical community and mainstream media began advising people to stop consuming the butter, lard, and bacon they'd been eating for centuries, replacing them with bread, pasta, margarine, low-fat dairy, and vegetable oil. It was a dietary shift that was ultimately codified by the U.S. government in the late 1970s.

How Nutritional Guidelines Have Decimated Public Health

In 1977, the U.S. released the first national dietary guidelines to urge Americans to cut back on fat intake.[27] In a radical departure from the prevailing diet of the time, the guidelines suggested Americans eat a diet high in grains and low in fat, with industrially processed vegetables oils taking the place of most animal fats.

According to research by Zoë Harcombe, Ph.D., published in the journal *Open Heart*, there was never any scientific basis for the recommendations to cut fat from the U.S. diet.[28] Dr. Harcombe and colleagues examined the evidence from randomized controlled trials (RCTs)—the gold standard of scientific research—available to the U.S. and U.K. regulatory committees at the time the guidelines were implemented. Six dietary trials involving 2,467 men were available, but there were no differences in all-cause mortality and only nonsignificant differences in heart-disease mortality resulting from the dietary interventions.

As noted in *Open Heart*, "Recommendations were made for 276 million people following secondary studies of 2467 males, which reported identical all-cause mortality. RCT evidence did not support the introduction of dietary fat guidelines."

Despite the lack of evidence to support them, the guidelines were quite extreme, calling for Americans to reduce overall fat consumption to 30 percent of total energy intake and limit saturated fat consumption to just 10 percent of total energy. The war on fat was on, and it has prevailed to this day: even as recently as December 2015, when the U.S. Department of Agriculture (USDA) released its most recent nutritional guidelines, cautions on saturated fat were still strongly worded, with Americans advised to "consume less than 10 percent of calories per day from saturated fats."[29]

In all these years, that very recommendation has actually fueled the problem it aimed to treat. No one knows for sure just how many premature deaths have resulted from this low-fat diet recommendation, but my guess is that this number is easily into the hundreds of millions.

THE LOW DIETARY FAT EXPERIMENT HAS BEEN A MISERABLE FAILURE

Ever since Ancel Keys catalyzed the shift to a low-fat diet in the 1950s, Americans have dutifully reduced their intake of animal fats. The pace of the change picked up following the introduction of the USDA Dietary Guidelines in 1980 and the subsequent retooling of the food industry to produce low-fat foods, replacing healthy saturated fats like butter and lard with harmful trans fats, industrially processed vegetable oils, and lots of refined sugar. (Food manufacturers needed some way to make their products more crave-worthy despite the absence of the luscious taste of butter and lard, so they turned to ever-increasing amounts of sugar, which appears in a myriad of processed foods.)

Yet despite adherence to these supposedly "healthy" guidelines, U.S. public health has declined precipitously, as evidenced by trends in the following areas:

- **Diabetes**

    In 1978, 5.19 million Americans had been di-agnosed with diabetes, according to the Centers for Disease Control. By 2013, it was 22.3 million—more than quadruple the number of people diagnosed with this deadly disease in just 35 years.[30]

- **Obesity**

    According to the National Health and Nutrition Examination Survey, from 1976 to 1980, 16.4 percent of adults were obese (defined as a BMI over 30) or extremely obese (BMI over 35). The latest numbers available at the time of this writing, from the *Journal of the American Medical Association*, put that total at more than 45.6 percent obese or extremely obese.[31] Whereas in the 1970s only one in about six people was obese, now nearly one out of two adults are afflicted.

- **Cancer**

    Obesity is a major risk factor in many cancers. In 1975, the rate of new cancer diagnoses was roughly 400 people out of every 100,000;[32] the estimated number of new cases of cancer in 2016 was nearly 449 people out of every 100,000—a statistically significant increase.[33]

- **Heart disease**

    Heart disease is also associated with obesity. Death rates from heart disease have declined since their peak in the 1950s, although much of this is due to advances in medical treatment, not improvements in health.

The prevalence of heart disease is still high, and headed higher: In 2010, approximately 36.9 percent of Americans were living with some form of cardio-vascular disease, and the rates are expected to keep rising. A study published in *Circulation*, the journal of the American Heart Association, projects that by 2030, over 40 percent of the U.S. population will be living with cardiovascular disease.[34]

Once you understand the differences in how your body metabolizes sugars as opposed to fats, you will be able to follow the money to get a clear picture of how these flawed guidelines have contributed to this huge decline in public health.

Remember, your body is designed to run much more efficiently on fats than on sugar. By eating more sugar and nonfiber carbs, which rapidly convert to sugar, you generate far more tissue-damaging free radicals than when you are primarily burning fat for fuel. Although free radicals do confer some important health benefits, when you overconsume sugar and nonfiber carbs you tip the balance of free radicals in your body in an unhealthy direction. This imbalance then creates a cascade of tissue, protein, cell membrane, and genetic damage, paving the way for inflammation and disease.

It's not just physical health that has been hurt by the war on saturated fat. For decades now, Americans have been counseled by the government, their doctors, and the mainstream media that all they need to do to lose weight and be healthy is to eat less—particularly less saturated fat—and exercise more. The reality is that eating low-fat and high-carb foods makes it extremely difficult to lose weight.

In simple terms, when you eat carbohydrates, your pancreas secretes insulin. And the more insulin you have in your blood, the more signals your body gets to store fat. In other words, by following the present dietary advice that was officially codified by the government in 1977, we as a nation have been doing the very things that cause us to gain weight and keep it on.

So if you've gamely followed the USDA's nutritional guidelines and started loading up on bread, fat-free cereals, and skim milk while also hitting the gym a few times a week, and your excess weight not only hasn't budged but has increased, well, whose fault is that? According to all the conventional sources of nutritional guidance, the fault is yours.

The assumption is that you must not have been trying hard enough, or you weren't doing it right. Of course, this is demoralizing. One of my primary intentions in creating MMT and writing this book is to show you that you absolutely do have the power to lose weight and restore your own health.

WHAT DOES THE SCIENCE SAY?

The ubiquitous story line in the media and the governmental public health agencies hasn't evolved much past Ancel Keys's observations in the early 1950s: avoid saturated fats because they raise your LDL cholesterol, which will ultimately clog your arteries and lead to heart disease.

The problem with this recommendation is that it's based only on a hypothesis, and worse yet, that hypothesis has never been proven. In fact, numerous studies over the decades have carefully examined the supposed link between saturated fats and heart disease and found it flawed.

Six major clinical trials on saturated fat have been used to support the assumption that saturated fats cause heart disease. In reality, however, none of them actually showed that eating fewer saturated fats would prevent heart disease and lengthen your life. In fact, none of these trials showed that restricting saturated fats reduced total mortality:

- The Oslo Study (1968) found eating a diet low in saturated fats and high in polyunsaturated fats had no influence on rates of sudden death.[35]

- The L.A. Veterans Study (1969) found no significant difference between rates of sudden death or heart attack among men eating a mostly animal-foods diet and those eating a high–vegetable oil diet. However, more noncardiac deaths, including from cancer, were seen in the vegetable oil group.[36]

- The Minnesota Coronary Survey (1968), a study funded by the National Institutes of Health, shows that more than four years of eating a low–saturated fat, high-PUFA diet led to no reduction in cardiovascular events, cardiovascular deaths, or total deaths.[37]

- The Finnish Mental Hospital Study (1968) found a reduction in heart disease among men following a low–saturated fat, high-PUFA diet, but no significant reduction was seen among women.[38]

- The London Soybean Oil Trial (1968) reported no difference in heart attack rate between men following a diet low in saturated fats and high in soybean oil and those following an ordinary diet.[39]

- The U.S. Multiple Risk Factor Intervention Trial (1982) compared mortality rates and eating habits of over 12,000 men, and its finding that people who ate a low–saturated fat and low-cholesterol diet had a marginal reduction in coronary heart disease was widely publicized. However, their mortality from all causes was higher, although this statistic received little coverage.[40]

More recently, three meta-analyses that collectively included data on hundreds of thousands of people have found that there is no difference in the risks of heart disease and stroke between people with the lowest and highest intakes of fat.[41, 42, 43] (Meta-analysis is a statistical technique for combining the findings from a selection of independent studies.)

And some research has found that replacing saturated animal fats with industrially processed omega-6 vegetable fats is linked to an *increased* risk of death among patients with heart disease. A *British Medical Journal* study published in 2013[44] included 458 men with a history of heart problems who were divided into two groups. One group reduced saturated fats to less than 10 percent of their energy intake and increased omega-6 fats from safflower oils to 15 percent of their energy intake. The control group continued to eat whatever they wanted. After 39 months:

- The omega-6 linoleic acid group had a 17 percent higher risk of dying from heart disease during the study period, compared with 11 percent among the control group.

- The omega-6 group also had a higher risk of all-cause mortality.

Another study published in the *British Medical Journal* in 2013[45] found that replacing saturated animal fats with industrially processed omega-6 vegetable fats is linked to an increased risk of death among patients with heart disease.

The Truth about Saturated Fat

Part of the enormous confusion about the dangers associated with saturated fats is related to their effect on LDL cholesterol, often referred to as "bad" cholesterol. But it's important to understand that when you hear the terms *LDL* and *HDL*, they're both referring to lipoproteins, which are simply proteins that carry cholesterol. LDL stands for low-density lipoprotein, while HDL stands for high-density lipoprotein.

HDL cholesterol is actually linked to a lower risk of heart disease, which is why measurements of total cholesterol are useless when it comes to measuring your risk. In fact, if your total cholesterol is "high" because you have a lot of HDL, it's no indication of increased heart risks; rather, it's likely protective.

Saturated fats have been shown to actually raise protective HDL cholesterol while also increasing LDL. The latter isn't necessarily bad either once you understand that there are different types of LDL:

- Small, dense LDL cholesterol
- Large, fluffy LDL cholesterol

Research has confirmed that large, fluffy LDL particles do not contribute to heart disease. The small, dense LDL particles, however, are easily oxidized, which may trigger heart disease. This is because the small, dense LDL penetrates your arterial wall more easily, so it contributes to the buildup of plaque in your arteries. Synthetic trans fat also increases small, dense LDL. Saturated fat, on the other hand, increases large, fluffy—and benign—LDL.

People with high levels of small, dense LDL have triple the heart disease risk of people with high levels of large, fluffy LDL.[46] And here's another fact that might blow your mind: eating saturated fat may change the small, dense LDL in your body into the healthier large, fluffy LDL![47, 48] Also important, research has shown that small, dense LDL particles are increased by eating refined sugar and carbohydrates, such as bread, bagels and soda.[49] Together, refined sugar and carbs do far more harm to your body than saturated fat ever could.

Based on what we know now about saturated fats, the irony is that they are actually necessary to promote health and prevent disease. Indeed, it's now known that saturated fats provide a number of important health benefits, including the following:

- Providing building blocks for cell membranes, hormones, and hormone-like substances
- Mineral absorption, such as calcium
- Acting as carriers for important fat-soluble vitamins A, D, E, and K
- Conversion of carotene into vitamin A
- Helping lower cholesterol levels (palmitic and stearic acids)
- Acting as antiviral agent (caprylic acid)
- Optimal fuel for your brain when fats are converted to ketones

- Helping you feel full and satisfied—meaning you're less likely to feel the need to snack on processed foods that may be high in flavor but low in nutrients

- Modulating genetic regulation and helping prevent cancer (butyric acid)

- Increasing your LDL levels, but this is largely an increase in large fluffy particles that are not associated with an increased risk of heart disease

- Boosting your HDL levels, which more than compensates for any increase in LDL

- Serving to fuel mitochondria and produce far fewer free radicals than carbs

The research has spelled out loud and clear that saturated fats are beneficial for human health. Most of us need to radically increase the healthy fat in our diet—this includes not only saturated fat but also monounsaturated fats (from avocados and certain nuts) and omega-3 fats—while severely limiting refined vegetable oils and even naturally occurring omega-6 fats (found in nuts and seeds).

If this sounds like a lot to remember, just hold on to this: for optimal health, eat real food—this means plenty of saturated fats and little to no refined fats, especially refined vegetable oils. Again, I will cover diet specifics in much more detail in Part II of this book.

CHAPTER 2

WHY YOU NEED MITOCHONDRIAL METABOLIC THERAPY (MMT)

The nutritional plan that I have developed—and that I outline in the second half of this book—is not for everyone. If you are merely looking for a way to upgrade your nutrition and improve your overall health with smart but quick fixes like making tweaks to the percentage of carbs, proteins, and fats you eat, and substituting nutrient-dense whole foods for foods with low nutritional value, you can easily do that by reviewing the Nutritional Plan on the right side of the home page on mercola. com or by reading my last book, *Effortless Healing*. But if you are facing serious health challenges, or if you are basically healthy now but want to *supercharge* your health, I wrote this book on MMT for you.

WHY MITOCHONDRIAL METABOLIC THERAPY?

As I've already stressed, optimally functioning mitochondria are absolutely vital to your overall health. You have between 80 and 2,000 mitochondria in nearly all of your cells and they generate around 90 percent of the energy you need to survive and stay healthy. When mitochondrial function is impaired—as it so easily is when you eat a typical American low-fat, high-carb, highly processed diet—this disrupts normal metabolic signaling, which in turn damages cellular and mitochondrial DNA or causes a defect in the ability to repair damage from other sources, such as environmental radiation.

To enable your body to prevent and fight cancer and most all major diseases, you have to take extraordinary care of your mitochondria. And the primary way to optimize, repair, and regenerate your mitochondria is to provide them with the best possible fuel. That's where Mitochondrial Metabolic Therapy comes in.

Rather than seeking to control the symptoms of chronic diseases, MMT seeks to heal the root cause of chronic disease and aging—the integrity, or lack thereof, of the mitochondria themselves.

The Difference between MMT and the Atkins and Paleo Diets

While I believe MMT is the best food plan to optimize mitochondrial function, many other popular diets are similar in some aspects to MMT—yet there are many key differences. These diets are:

- **Atkins:** A true nutritional pioneer, Dr. Robert Atkins began spreading the word in the 1970s that our carb-laden diets weren't healthy, and spread it did. His first book, **Dr. Atkins' Diet Revolution,** sold over 15 million copies, and more than 30 million Americans followed his low-carb diet plan. I use the term **low carb** very specifically, because his advice was focused more on reducing carbs than it was on burning fat.

Atkins introduced the term "ketosis" to the American public, but because of the word's similarity to "ketoacidosis"—a potentially life-threatening condition that can occur in type 1 diabetics—he quickly backed away from emphasizing fat as a preferred source of fuel. Instead he took aim at bread and pasta as our primary dietary villains.

Atkins was very close to espousing an ideal diet. He certainly broke new ground, especially in the minds of the public. His important role in public education was indisputable. But there were a couple of major flaws in his diet plan:

Primary focus is on weight loss. The Atkins Diet became as popular as it did because it promised quick and effortless weight loss. Although shedding excess pounds can potentially benefit health in many ways, weight (especially fat) loss in and of itself is only a side effect of MMT. Although I admit that fat loss is a welcome side effect for most people, the true aim of MMT is to heal your metabolism at the cellular level and ward off the development of most common chronic diseases and premature aging—a far more ambitious goal than simply fitting into your skinny jeans.

Too much protein. Because the war on fat was in full swing, the Atkins Diet was painted as a dangerous fad, and ketosis was viewed as an aberrant and undesirable metabolic state. Despite Atkins's advice to consume leafy green vegetables, many followers relied too heavily on protein to replace the calories that otherwise would have come from carbs, resulting in a stereotype of his followers bingeing on steak, eggs, cheese, and bacon. As I discuss in Chapter 4, a high-protein diet is even more dangerous than a high-carb diet, and the average American is already consuming far too much protein, a problem I've addressed with MMT.

No attention to food quality. Perhaps most importantly, Atkins did not counsel his followers to avoid low-quality foods, whether that was feedlot beef, pasteurized dairy, or refined vegetable oils. While his focus on macronutrients (which is a fancy way of referring to broad categories of food, such as carb, fat, or protein) was on the right track, the individual foods within those macronutrient categories were inherently dangerous. As a result, the Atkins diet was pro-inflammatory and ultimately detrimental to mitochondrial health. Also, many Atkins products were highly processed bars and shakes that relied on artificial sweeteners—decidedly not real food.

May or may not result in a shift to fat burning. Although it was a low-carb diet, the excess protein most people consumed while following the Atkins plan was enough to keep many of them from making the metabolic switch to fat burning. This process that can take weeks, if not months, and it generally needs at least some period of careful blood glucose monitoring and ketone level checks to truly confirm that you have made the transition to burning fat. (I will walk you through this process in the chapters to come.)

- **Paleo:** Based on the eating habits of our Paleolithic ancestors, who ate primarily vegetables, fruit, nuts, roots, and meat, the Paleo diet is very clear about eliminating grains and legumes but doesn't place hard limits on high-net-carb vegetables, fruits, and sugars such as honey or coconut sugar.

  The Paleo diet is wildly popular with good reason. It takes us back to the basics; it refocuses the diet on fresh, whole, unprocessed, "real" food as the foundational first step in optimizing health and addressing just about any health condition. While the standard Paleo diet can be a healthful way of eating, and is light years ahead of the standard American diet, it too has weaknesses or flaws that make it less than ideal:

  Too heavy an emphasis on protein. Protein is freely substituted for carbs as being a healthy choice. The Paleo diet calls for about 38 percent protein and 39 percent fat,[1] which may actually be too much protein and not enough fat for optimal health. As you will learn later, protein levels closer to 10 percent during nutritional ketosis is far more optimal. They can increase to higher percentages, especially for those individuals still in the midst of the reproductive and athletic performance years, but those pursuing optimizing their biology would not want higher levels for extended periods.

  Not enough caution regarding seafood. The Paleo diet includes lots of fish and other seafood on a regular basis, and this appears to be reasonable as docosahexaenoic acid (DHA), a type of omega-3 fat found in fish, is clearly one of the most important and essential nutrients for your health. But there is one important caveat: as a result of industrial pollution made up of a variety of toxins, including mercury, PCBs, and dioxin, it is difficult to find seafood that is toxin free. For this reason, I only recommend seafood that is high in healthy fats while being minimally exposed to toxic contaminants. I offer specific suggestions on how to find that, as well as how to avoid being duped by deceptively marketed seafood, in Chapter 5.

Too many starches and sugars (net carbs). Even though sweet potatoes and fruits—two popular foods on the Paleo plan—are whole foods, they still raise glucose and trigger an insulin reaction, especially when you are seeking to make the transition from sugar to fat burning. This is likely to become a nonissue once you are fat adapted, which means you are able to burn fat rather than carbs as your primary fuel. A central goal of MMT is to lower blood glucose levels, and therefore insulin levels, so that insulin resistance can resolve.

In many ways, MMT can be seen as an important refinement of Paleo, taking the whole-food, no-grain foundation and building upon it by emphasizing high-quality fats, keeping nonfiber carbs to about 50 grams a day (or less), and avoiding even natural sugars such as dates (except for the sweeteners that I will cover later).

The problem here is obvious. On the one hand, your mitochondria are vital to your overall health—they generate ATP and control apoptosis (programmed cell death) as well as autophagy and mitophagy, which clear out unhealthy cells and mitochondria before they can contribute to the processes that lead to the development of chronic disease. On the other hand, your mitochondria are prime sites for ROS production *and* free radical damage because they contain two cell membranes, an inner and outer one, both of which are extremely vulnerable to damage.

The question, then, is how to manufacture ATP as efficiently as possible in order to optimize your health and longevity while sidestepping the problems that arise from a lifetime of eating food that produces an excess of free radicals when it is metabolized.

The good news is that using ketones for energy creates significantly fewer free radicals than sugar. Because ketones simply burn far cleaner than sugar, they cause far less oxidative damage, which is one of the core reasons why a fat-burning food plan such as MMT is so powerful.

It's important to note that the biggest impact on lowering exposure to oxidative damage comes when you keep your blood glucose levels low, as evidenced by Dr. Seyfried's work to establish the Glucose Ketone Index (GKI).[2] This is why monitoring your blood glucose levels is an integral part of MMT (which I cover in depth in chapters 6 and 7).

ADDITIONAL BENEFITS OF MITOCHONDRIAL METABOLIC THERAPY

Beyond feeding your body a cleaner fuel and naturally limiting ROS generation, MMT provides a host of physiological benefits. When you take an objective look at them, I believe you too will see that following its guidelines is one of the best choices you can make for your health. These benefits include:

Mental Clarity

Your brain cannot function properly without healthy fats. Because your brain is 60 percent fat, eating healthy fats that build biologically responsive cellular membranes is crucial for optimal brain function. By contrast, overindulging on sugar and grains eventually leads to neural impairment and damage, in part because it blocks insulin's ability to regulate normal cellular activities.[3]

The connection between sugar and Alzheimer's disease was first made in 2005, when the disease was tentatively dubbed "type 3 diabetes." Previous research has also shown that people with diabetes have a twofold increased risk of developing Alzheimer's disease. It's little wonder, then, that MMT, which will make it easy for you to transition to fat burning while also removing nearly all high-net-carb foods from your diet until you are able to burn fat as your primary fuel, will produce a noticeable boost in your mental clarity. This approach improves your brain function today and reduces your risk of dementia tomorrow.

I never could have written this book as quickly as I did without the clearheadedness MMT has provided. In fact, I have personally experienced such an uptick in creativity and cognition that I need Google Keep—a note-taking app that you can use on your computer or device—to quickly and easily capture my thoughts and ideas and then store them in a searchable way.

Freedom from Cravings

Processed food, with all its chemical additives, added sugars, and refined oils and carbohydrates, is extremely addictive. This has been demonstrated by a number of studies spanning decades of research[4, 5] and is no accident. The food industry employs teams of scientists who scheme to improve the "mouthfeel" of fake, processed food. They do this to maximize food cravings so you will continue to come back for more even when your body doesn't need nourishment.

When you burn sugar for your primary fuel, metabolic pathways are activated that cause you to crave replenishment by driving your blood sugar down after a few hours without sugar, which keeps you on a hamster wheel of hunger, cravings, and crashes.

Fat, by contrast, is naturally satiating, meaning it leaves your belly full and satisfies your desire for food. And when you make the switch to burning fat as a predominant fuel, you can access the tens of thousands of calories[6] that are stored within your own body fat—calories that are largely unavailable to you if you are burning sugar as your primary fuel. As a result, you will find that you can go for long periods of time without even thinking about food, let alone having to deal with specific cravings—these will disappear once your body has adapted to burning fat for fuel.

One note: If you notice that you're craving fat, most likely you haven't been taking in quite enough fat. That's one reason I love "fat bombs"—tasty treats that consist primarily of coconut oil or other healthy fats—as they are simple, delicious, and portable ways to take in a couple of teaspoons of fat. (See page 260 for online resources for numerous fat bomb recipes.)

An Anticancer Strategy

In recent years, scientists have come to realize that it's not genetic mutations that cause cancer. We now know that *mitochondrial damage happens first.*

Mitochondrial dysfunction produces reactive oxygen species, mentioned earlier, which in turn can cause DNA mutations, making the mutations an effect of abnormal respiration. The ROS then further damage the mitochondria, and thus respiration, creating a vicious cycle.

This understanding has taken decades to piece together. In 1924, Dr. Otto Warburg, who went on to win the Nobel Prize in Physiology or Medicine in 1931, made the discovery—now known as the Warburg effect—that cancer cells have a fundamentally different energy metabolism compared to healthy cells. The Warburg effect tells us that most of the mitochondria in cancer cells are dysfunctional and can't use oxygen to burn fuel efficiently—they lack the metabolic flexibility to metabolize fats. For this reason, they rely on fermenting ever-increasing amounts of glucose in their cytoplasm (instead of oxidizing it in their mitochondria), a far less efficient way of obtaining energy called lactic acid fermentation.

Thanks to the work of Dr. Peter Pedersen from Johns Hopkins, we also know that a universal characteristic of cancer cells is that they have a radically reduced number of fully functional mitochondria.

Dr. Thomas N. Seyfried, an internationally known researcher on the link between metabolism and disease and author of the 2012 landmark book *Cancer as a Metabolic Disease*, puts another nail in the coffin of the "cancer is a genetic disease" theory by explaining in his work that there are some cancers that have no genetic mutations, but still rely on fermentation rather than respiration for their energy. And that there are some known carcinogens, such as arsenic and asbestos, that do not directly cause genetic mutation. Rather, they damage the mitochondrial function of respiration, which then produces the Warburg effect and cancer.

Seyfried also elucidates that the proliferation of cancer cells disappears when the nucleus of a tumor cell is transferred to a normal cell that contains normal mitochondria. Further, the abnormal growth and metastatic behavior of breast cancer cells disappear when mitochondria from healthy cells replace the abnormal breast cancer mitochondria, despite the continued presence of the tumor nucleus.

These and many other findings indicate that cancer cannot be a genetic disease.

What all this means it that when you remove processed foods, sugar, grains, and high-net-carb fuels from your diet, you essentially stress cancer cells by depriving them of their preferred metabolic fuel.[7]

For this reason, I believe MMT is one of the most powerful cancer prevention strategies available because it optimizes your mitochondrial function, and as a result, the mitochondria are less easily damaged and the genetic mutations that can lead to cancer are radically reduced.

MMT also has enormous benefit if you are already dealing with cancer. Making the switch to burning ketone bodies will deprive cancer cells of their primary fuel, which then causes them adverse stress. At the same time, your healthy cells are given a cleaner and more ideal fuel, which lowers oxidative stress, conserves antioxidants, and optimizes mitochondrial function. The sum effect is that healthy cells begin to thrive while cancer cells must struggle to survive.

Microbiome Changes

Recent estimates suggest your body houses some 30 trillion bacteria[8] and about 1 quadrillion viruses (bacteriophages). In essence, we're little more than walking microbe colonies.

These organisms perform a wide variety of functions, including:

- Assisting in the digestion of food

- Regulating the enteric nervous system, which rules the digestive tract

- Orchestrating the immune response

- Helping modulate many aspects of inflammation

- Playing a large role in brain and mental health, as the gut and the brain are intricately connected

Emerging science also shows that your microbiome can be rapidly altered, for better or worse, based on factors such as diet, lifestyle, and chemical exposures, including over-the-counter medications and prescribed antibiotics, as well as those introduced into the food supply that have been widely fed to the animals we consume.

The MMT food plan up-regulates, modifies, and improves the quality of your gut microbiome. It cuts out known microbiome disruptors such as various sugars, processed foods, and artificial sweeteners.

Weight Loss without Deprivation

When your body burns glucose as its primary fuel, your ability to access and burn body fat is inhibited. With an ever-present supply of carbs, your liver down-regulates the entire fat-burning process because you are not regularly cycling between feast-and-famine modes. Excess glucose is also stored as fat—unlike ketones, which are excreted through the urine if they aren't taken up by cells.

Fat cells produce their own hormones, including leptin. This may seem like a good thing, but when you consistently consume too much sugar and store more fat, your leptin levels rise and the leptin receptors become less sensitive and eventually more resistant to healthy levels of leptin. For this reason, when you burn glucose as your primary fuel, your fat cells trap you in a vicious cycle of storing more fat and becoming less and less adept at burning the fat you already have.

In this way, hormones and the communication between them play an important role in both weight control *and* your urge to eat, and even what you crave. And those hormones are determined by the foods you eat. As Dr. Rosedale puts it, "You eat today to control the hormones that will tell your cells what to eat tomorrow."[9]

Which is precisely how MMT works. It uses food intake to modulate the levels of your hormones—including leptin and insulin—that influence your weight, thereby directing your body to *burn* fat, not *store* it. It also removes the sources of sugars from your diet, which helps free you from that vicious cycle. As a result, your body will release its hold on your excess weight. And it does this *without* the stereotypical hunger pangs and cravings that accompany most weight-loss diets.

Greatly Improved Energy

MMT improves the mitochondria you already have and stimulates the creation of new mitochondria. Since mitochondria are the primary sources of energy production in your body, MMT also produces a palpable uptick in energy.

Because your body will produce fewer destructive ROS as it metabolizes ketone bodies instead of sugar, you will have to spend less cellular energy on mopping up rogue free radicals—this also contributes to the net energy gain MMT can provide.

Increased Insulin Sensitivity

Any meal or snack high in net carbs typically generates a rapid rise in blood glucose. To compensate for this, your pancreas secretes insulin into your bloodstream, which in turn lowers your blood sugar to keep it in normal ranges because excess glucose is toxic to your cells. Insulin is also very efficient at lowering blood sugar by inhibiting the production of glucose by your liver (a process known as gluconeogenesis).

Unfortunately, if you consume a diet consistently high in sugar and grains, your blood glucose levels will be correspondingly high, and over time your insulin receptors become "desensitized" to insulin, requiring more and more insulin to get the job done. This is referred to as insulin resistance. Approximately 45 percent of Americans now have some degree of insulin resistance, and over time this number is expected to rise.

Because MMT does not include foods that your body can easily convert to glucose—such as grains, sugars, and high-net-carb foods—it keeps your blood glucose levels low, which in turn keeps your insulin levels low. Lowering glucose and insulin gives your insulin receptors a chance to regain their sensitivity.

Reducing Inflammation

Sugar fans the flames of inflammation in your body, as it is a dirty fuel that was never intended to be our primary fuel. Using sugar for energy produces 30 to 40 percent more ROS than burning fat.

Omega-6 oils, particularly those that are heavily refined and easily oxidized, tend to be highly inflammatory. In MMT, you will limit your consumption of these bad fats and get most of what you need from oil-rich foods containing healthier oils. Increasing your consumption of omega-3 fats will improve the ratio of omega-6 to omega-3 fats, which you will learn is important to cellular health.

Saturated fats, on the other hand, are not oxidized as easily as oils because they don't have double bonds that can be damaged through oxidation. MMT prioritizes getting your fats from healthful sources of saturated and monounsaturated fats and significantly reduces your omega-6 oil consumption. It's no surprise, then, that research shows that low-carb diets tend to reduce levels of systemic inflammation.[10]

Self-Eating: Autophagy and Mitophagy

The term *autophagy* means "self-eating," and refers to the processes by which your body cleans out accumulated debris, including toxins, and recycles damaged cell components. Autophagy occurs within your mitochondria. When the entire mitochondria is digested and removed, the process is called mitophagy.

Both these processes are incredibly important contributors to your health—in fact, the 2016 Nobel Prize in Medicine went to Yoshinori Ohsumi, a researcher who discovered the mechanisms that drive autophagy.[11]

When autophagy and mitophagy are inhibited through poor diet, excess ROS, and high levels of inflammation, the damaged mitochondria linger in the cell, emitting pro-inflammatory molecules and generally accelerating the aging process. So autophagy and mitophagy play an important role in controlling the amount of inflammation in your body and help slow down the aging process.

These processes are largely controlled by the mechanistic (formerly known as mammalian) target of rapamycin (mTOR)—a primary metabolic regulatory pathway that I cover more extensively in Chapter 3. When mTOR is activated, it fuels growth and regeneration, and its activity can enhance cellular maintenance and repair. MMT inhibits (down-regulates) this mTOR pathway, and as a result, stimulates autophagy and mitophagy.

Mitochondrial Biogenesis
(The Creation of New Mitochondria)

Biogenesis is the process by which new healthy mitochondria can be duplicated. When it comes to maintaining optimal biological functioning and good health, the more healthy mitochondria you have, the better off you will be.

Research has shown that shifting to a fat-burning diet spurs mitochondrial biogenesis—at least in a rodent model.[12] On a fat-burning diet, mitochondria are not kept busy fighting off free radicals (since fat burning creates far fewer harmful reactive oxygen species than burning sugar). The beneficial effect is that mitochondria now have more energy to focus on the processes involved in creating more—and healthier—mitochondria. In a sense, your mitochondria become supercharged!

THE INFLUENCE OF KETONES

When I say that you "burn fat" on MMT, what I really mean is that you burn ketones. Ketones are also referred to as *ketone bodies*, an old-school biochemistry term. The terms *ketones* and *ketone bodies* are interchangeable and often used in place of each other. In this book, I'll stick with *ketones*.

Ketones are water-soluble energy molecules that are made by mitochondria in your liver from dietary or stored fats and are used as an alternative fuel to glucose. Because they are water soluble, ketones don't need carrier proteins to travel in the blood stream; they pass easily through your cell membranes and even cross the blood-brain barrier.[13]

In fact, ketones are a brilliant biological adaptation that provides a critically important fuel for your body and brain during times of food scarcity. Without ketones, you wouldn't be able to live more than a few weeks without food. It was previously thought that the brain only used sugar for fuel, and many health professionals and organizations are still espousing this outdated notion today, but the late George Cahill disproved that 50 years ago.[14] The truth is that your body is exquisitely wired to fuel your brain because your brain consumes up to 20 percent of your total caloric intake. The ability of your brain to transition to ketone metabolism extends the survival of a fasting human from a few weeks to over a month. The longest recorded human fast was a year and 17 days—only the efficiency of ketones would allow such a remarkable feat.

Ketones are also an important component of MMT, as their presence indicates that you are burning fat as your primary fuel instead of glucose.

There are three different types of ketones, including:

- Acetoacetate, which is a precursor to the other two forms of ketones and which is excreted in urine

- Beta-hydroxybutyrate (BHB), the most abundant ketone, which circulates in the blood and is used for energy

- Acetone, which is exhaled through your breath

Ketones—Villains or Heroes?

Sadly, to this day there is serious confusion in the public and even among most medical professionals about ketones. This confusion is regarding the difference between nutritional ketosis and diabetic ketoacidosis. Although they both share part of one word, *keto-*, they are two entirely different metabolic states.

Nutritional ketosis is the state you achieve when you enter a fat-burning state. It is an exceptionally healthy way to create the conditions your body needs to stay healthy and age well. In nutritional ketosis, blood ketone levels are typically between 0.5 and 3 mmol/liter and rarely exceed 6 to 8 mmol/liter. Blood glucose levels also lowered to healthy levels of 70 mg/dl or less.

On the other extreme, diabetic ketoacidosis is a life-threatening symptom of uncontrolled diabetes and can be fatal if not properly treated. In contrast, ketone levels in diabetic ketoacidosis are typically over 20 mmol/liter. The true danger of diabetic ketoacidosis is that glucose levels are also very high, at least 250 mg/dl, although they can even exceed 400 mg/dl! This results in a severe metabolic acidosis and secondary severe dehydration that require intensive medical management.

Ketoacidosis occurs in type 1 diabetes because insulin levels are very low. Because you need insulin to suppress glucose production in the liver, it continues to make glucose even when you aren't eating. High glucose should turn off ketone production, but again, the lack of insulin means there is no signal to stop making ketones. Since there's plenty of glucose available, the ketones are not used up by the brain as fuel. They pile up and cause a metabolic acidosis.

By contrast, in nutritional ketosis, unless you have been fasting for a long time, there is still enough insulin present to suppress liver glucose production. Glucose levels drop as you lower your carb intake and the brain burns off the ketones you make, so high levels never occur.

So, it is the simultaneous metabolic effect of very high ketones, very high glucose, and dehydration that causes the life-threatening metabolic issues associated with diabetic ketoacidosis. This condition can't exist in nutritional ketosis, but that's still where many conventional doctors are stuck in their outdated thinking.

Dr. Atkins was the first physician to introduce ketosis to the public as a desirable effect of lowering carbohydrates in the diet, but the term "nutritional ketosis" had not yet been coined. Because of this confusion, as well as the demonization of fats, he encountered resistance to using the term in his books, which is why he ended up emphasizing the low-carb facet of his diet rather than its fat-burning benefits.

Research since then (Dr. Atkins died in 2004) has clarified the difference in the impacts between unhealthy fats and healthy fats. Thankfully in the 21st century there have been reams of published studies supporting the metabolic benefits of nutritional ketosis. These, coupled with the testimonials of those experiencing these benefits, are starting to lessen the confusion on this issue, allowing many more health care practitioners and even conventional doctors—heretofore AWOL on nutritional matters—open to the use of this diet intervention.

Why Do We Even Make Ketones?

Ketones weren't discovered until the late 1800s when they made an undignified debut in the urine of patients with uncontrolled diabetes (as diabetic ketoacidosis).[15] Within a few decades researchers had also learned that there was a positive aspect of ketone production.

Whenever your supply of carbohydrates from food is low or nonexistent, even after just a couple of days or so, your body is able to convert fat to ketones. This metabolic flexibility is an important reason why the human race has been able to survive; it helps us adapt to a wide variety of food sources.

In addition to allowing us to survive periods of food scarcity, ketones provide many powerful health benefits:

- When your cells burn ketones for fuel, far fewer ROS are produced than when you burn glucose. In essence, ketones are a much "cleaner" energy source than glucose, meaning that they result in far less mitochondrial damage than occurs when glucose is used as fuel.

- If you switch to burning fats (including ketones), you decrease the amount of sugar available to cancer cells. You also reduce the amount of ROS your cells are exposed to, making it less likely that cancer will form in the first place.

- The most abundant ketone, beta-hydroxybutyrate (BHB), carries out a variety of signaling functions that can ultimately affect gene expression.[16]

- Ketones play an important role in reducing inflammation by reducing, or down-regulating, pro-inflammatory cytokines and increasing, or up-regulating, anti-inflammatory cytokines.[17]

- Ketones share a close structural similarity to branched-chain amino acids (BCAAs) and your body prefers them over BCAAs. That gives ketones a profoundly powerful protein-sparing effect, allowing you to consume lower quantities of protein while retaining or even building your muscle mass.[18] Additionally, BCAAs are a potent stimulus of the mTOR molecular signaling pathway, a very important metabolic pathway that is often overactive in disease states, including cancer. So when you maintain nutritional ketosis you also inhibit mTOR, and reduced activity here is associated with improvements in health span and longevity.[19] (However, mTOR has a positive role, especially in the young, as a potent stimulator of muscle protein synthesis. Many competitive athletes and bodybuilders seek to activate this pathway at the expense of the longevity-enhancing benefits of inhibiting mTOR.)[20]

- Studies suggest that ketones provide important protective benefits for brain cells that are exposed to hydrogen peroxide—a common presence in the brains of people with neurodegenerative diseases such as dementia and Alzheimer's disease.[21] Hydrogen peroxide converts to the dangerous hydroxyl free radical when your iron levels are high, as we will discuss in Chapter 4. So you will get more benefit from ketones when your iron levels are optimized.

- Ketones up-regulate (increase) mitochondrial biogenesis in your brain[22]—meaning that they help your body improve its capacity to produce more energy by increasing the number of mitochondria.

- Anecdotal reports suggest that in some people, fasting or transitioning to a low-carb diet produces feelings of mild euphoria, suggesting that ketones play a role in promoting the experience of well-being.[23]

Despite these benefits, simply producing enough ketones to officially be in nutritional ketosis is not the main goal of MMT. Eating a supremely healthful diet that keeps your body in a fat-burning state is the ultimate goal. This is why you won't hear me refer to MMT as a "ketogenic diet"—a term often used to describe similar high-fat, low-carb diets—because that phrase implies that the whole purpose of the diet is to have as many ketones around as possible. That is not the case. As I have mentioned, the end goals of MMT are to optimize your mitochondria, reduce free radical damage, and address the root of disease. Ketones are a means to these, not an end.

Improved Quality of Life and Prolonged Survival In a Case of Pediatric Brain Cancer

Miriam Kalamian has the most extensive experience of any clinician out there in applying the principles of MMT to the treatment of cancer. She helped edit most of this book, and I asked her to share her son's story, which catalyzed her drive to empower as many cancer patients as possible.

When my precious son, Raffi, was four years old, we discovered that he had a brain tumor. Stunned, my husband and I immediately agreed to start the standard of care: 14 months of weekly treatments with a combination of chemotherapy drugs. When that failed, Raffi's options were limited to other therapies with even less of a chance of response. Over the next year and a half, he endured high-risk surgeries, increasing hydrocephalus, and the side effects of the drugs he received through a clinical trial. Again and again, we experienced the disappointment of failed therapies, and it became clear that our young son was losing his hard-fought battle.

Now, at just seven years of age, his team was shuffling him into palliative care. The story could have ended there, except that one night as I was investigating one of the many drugs my son was receiving, I stumbled on Dr. Thomas Seyfried's groundbreaking research advancing his theory that cancer is a primarily a metabolic disease that can be managed with diet therapy. Could we manage Raffi's relentless disease without toxic drugs?

As thrilling as this possibility was to imagine, there were many challenges to overcome: First, I had no training in nutrition. Another broader issue was that there was no real precedent for the use of a high-fat, low-carb diet as a therapy for cancer. On the plus side, a team at Johns Hopkins with extensive experience in using this diet for treatment-resistant pediatric epilepsy had just published a new edition of a how-to book including "speculation" that a ketogenic diet might benefit those with brain cancer.

Then, on the Charlie Foundation website, I found some compassionate and keto-savvy parents willing to answer my many questions. Still, I never could have gone down this path without the encouragement of Raffi's local oncologist and pediatrician. Their support allowed us to overcome the intimidation and obstacles put in our path by his team of highly ranked specialists.

In the spring of 2007, my husband and I moved Raffi to a ketogenic diet armed with only this tiny toolkit. Following the model used in the epilepsy world, I chose to start him with a fast. It was a rough first day, mentally and physically, but thankfully kids are very metabolically flexible, much more so than most adults, and it wasn't long before Raffi was humming along on ketones and fats. And in fact, this seemingly harsh start was no rougher than the many days Raffi had spent dealing with the GI side effects of his drug therapies.

Amazingly, Raffi's symptoms began to improve almost immediately. He had more energy, could think more clearly, and even regained some of the vision that the tumor had robbed from him. We knew we were on the right track! It took some time and tweaking to get to a good place with this new way of eating, but we were generously rewarded for our efforts. Just three short months after starting the diet, Raffi's newest MRI scan clearly showed some shrinkage of the tumor mass.

This hit me like a ton of bricks: Why wasn't everyone given this life-changing information? A ketogenic diet is nothing more than a different mix of familiar foods, so why was there such pushback from the conventional medical and nutrition communities?

Raffi's success drove my desire to help others learn about this dietary option (as an adjunct to, not a substitute for, standard care). Within a few weeks, I had enrolled in a graduate program in nutrition, excited by the belief that I could then share what I was learning with people who were willing to modify their diet in exchange for a better quality of life—and perhaps even a longer life.

Raffi ultimately succumbed to his disease, but I never felt that the diet was a failure. During most of the six years he spent on a ketogenic diet, our family was devoted to enjoying the moment, which included an awesome five months spent camping on the Baja peninsula, "chillaxing" in the sun instead of being tied to the oncology clinic. These tangible results, along with the sense of empowerment and control the diet gave us in those years, continue to drive my passion to help others. The fact that I'm honoring Raffi with the work I do is a wonderful bonus.

I officially began my practice in 2010, and since that time I've guided hundreds of people with cancer through the transition to a therapeutic diet. Although many of these people experience what their oncologist views as "an amazing response to treatment," the diet remains woefully underutilized and mostly dismissed by a world that prides itself in sticking to "evidence-based" therapies even as millions die of this devastating disease. I truly believe in this diet, and that's why I was excited to add my insights and experiences to a book that offers such a clear path to better health.

CHAPTER 3

THE PROTEIN PARADOX

As I mentioned in the Introduction, Dr. Rosedale has been one of my primary nutritional mentors, and particularly in the last year or two as I've pieced together the understanding that was a catalyst for writing this book. I am grateful to him for helping me understand these important concepts, particularly in regard to the roles of protein and insulin on mitochondrial metabolic health.

Protein is essential for your health. It's a structural component of enzymes, cellular receptors, and signaling molecules, and it's the main building block for your muscles and bones. Proteins also perform transport carrier functions, and the amino acid components of proteins serve as precursors to hormones and vitamins.

When you consume more protein than your body needs, however, your kidneys are tasked with removing more nitrogen waste products from your blood. This added stress is one factor that can worsen kidney function if you already have kidney disease.[1] As with many areas in life, and contrary to the recommendations found in many popular diets such as Atkins and Paleo, more protein is not necessarily better. You *can* get too much of a good thing.

It's important to recognize that there is an upper limit to how much protein will actually benefit you. On average, Americans consume *far* more protein than they need, along with far too many carbohydrates and insufficient amounts of healthy fats. It's now clear that we need a complete realignment of the components of our diet.

To understand why eating too much protein is a bad idea, you need a basic understanding of the following concepts:

CALORIE RESTRICTION

For 60 years the gold standard in preserving health, extending life, and slowing down the aging process in animal studies has been calorie restriction, where you simply lower your caloric intake while still eating enough to prevent malnutrition. Calorie restriction is known to alter the expression of hundreds to thousands of genes. Some of these are related to longevity and some play a role in metabolism, cell growth, reproduction, immune response, and other important biological processes. These effects have been observed in a variety of species from worms and yeast to rats and fish, and there's strong evidence that suggests calorie restriction has a similar effect on the human life span as well.[2]

Despite its simplicity and proven merit, calorie restriction remains a strategy few people are willing to embrace. The good news is that eating a high-fat, adequate-protein, and low-carb diet allows you to reap the benefits of calorie restriction without deprivation or difficulty.

The research community has recently begun to tease out that it's not a lack of *total* calories that triggers the beneficial effects of energy-restricted diets. Instead, the latest science suggests that this phenomenon may actually result more from reduced protein intake—specifically the reduced intake of the amino acid methionine, high levels of which are found in meats.[3] To be clear, you do not want to eliminate methionine entirely, as methionine is a methyl donor for one of the most important antioxidants you have, glutathione. You just need to lower it.

Insulin

Insulin is an ancient hormone that is present in most biological life, from worms and flies all the way to humans. In humans, its prime role is to control nutrient storage—a way to carry energy forward during times of abundance to buffer those times when food is scarce. More specifically, its job is to help convert excess carbohydrates into fat.

It also plays a dual role in regard to aging. If your body perceives that food is abundant, insulin sends the all-clear signal to reproduce, and all processes are geared toward creating new life—and away from preserving your own.

On the other hand, if your body perceives a famine, an array of protective and regenerative mechanisms are switched on, ensuring our species's survival through lean times in order to fulfill the biological imperative to reproduce.

In general, the lower your average insulin level and the better your insulin receptor sensitivity, the slower the aging process. In fact, according to studies of the planet's oldest living people, lower insulin levels and higher insulin receptor sensitivity are associated with longer life.

Insulin-Like Growth Factor One (IGF-1)

Excess protein also stimulates the production of a hormone called insulin-like growth factor one, or IGF-1 for short. The name alone reveals much about the hormone; it is a close relative of insulin itself, and not surprisingly, it plays a somewhat similar role. The two hormones are so similar that they even cross-react with each other's receptors.

Human growth hormone (HGH) acts as a messenger for IGF-1. Once released by your pituitary, HGH stimulates the manufacture and release of IGF-1, which is responsible for most of the anabolic and growth effects attributed to HGH. Critically, IGF-1 tells your body to grow by instructing cells to reproduce. But this process, which results in a stronger organism, comes with a high price tag. Like insulin, IGF-1 is a powerful stimulus of aging, evidenced by studies showing that animals that produce less IGF-1 live significantly longer, less disease-ridden lives compared to those that produce high levels of the hormone.

Studies conducted on a community of people living in a remote corner of Ecuador who were afflicted with a rare form of dwarfism called Laron syndrome confirm the association between IGF-1 and disease.[4] Scientists around the world were shocked when it was reported that people with Laron syndrome lived long lives, virtually immune to diabetes and cancer.

After following 99 people with the syndrome for five years, researchers did not observe a single case of diabetes and recorded only one case of cancer—and the patient survived the disease. The researchers then compared these results to more than 1,000 normal-height relatives of Laron patients and found that the cancer death rate for these relatives was one in five. In addition, 5 percent of the relatives died from diabetes. Even though the Laron-syndrome community had a high prevalence of obesity, they were surprisingly insulin sensitive. These stunning findings were confirmed by studying a separate population with Laron syndrome living in Europe.

When researchers analyzed the blood of the Laron-syndrome patients, they were surprised to find high levels of HGH. But when they looked further they found the answer: a mutation in the receptor for HGH. In other words, the Laron patients were unable to respond to HGH by producing IGF-1. To most researchers, it was shocking in its own right that the lack of IGF-1 could have such a dramatic impact on two of the developed world's most pernicious and devastating diseases.

The Mammalian (or Mechanistic) Target of Rapamycin (mTOR)

mTOR, which I first described in Chapter 2, is a complex ancient protein that serves as your body's most important nutrient signaling pathway. It was only recently discovered during the process of developing the potent cancer drug rapamycin from a bacterium that was discovered on Easter Island in the late 1960s.[5] Most physicians learn nothing about this vital pathway during their training, but it is the key muscle-building mechanism in all mammals. When mTOR is not stimulated, it instructs the cell to turn on the array of repair and maintenance processes at its disposal, including autophagy (cleaning up cellular debris), DNA repair, and activating intracellular antioxidants and heat-shock proteins (HSPs). When it is activated, most typically by excess protein, it cues the cell to grow and proliferate; it also suppresses most cellular and mitochondrial repair and regeneration mechanisms.

If you maintain low levels of glucose, excess amino acids, insulin, and growth factors (like IGF-1), you will inhibit mTOR, thereby allowing the up-regulation of gene expression that promotes cellular and mitochondrial maintenance and repair. Hence your diet can have a profound influence on your overall health, possibly even your life span, and more importantly, your health span: the number of years that you live and are actually healthy.

Of all the nutrients that stimulate mTOR, amino acids—which are derived from protein—are the most potent. Stimulating mTOR by eating large amounts of protein is also one of the quickest ways to suppress cellular and mitochondrial autophagy, which prevents your body from effectively cleaning out debris and damaged cells. Even if you are optimizing everything you can to keep glucose and insulin levels low, eating excessive protein will still activate the mTOR pathway. If your goals are to treat disease and live long, doing this chronically is something you want to avoid.

Virtually all cancers are associated with mTOR activation, and inhibiting mTOR with drugs, such as rapamycin, for which mTOR is named, is a common and highly effective anticancer treatment. This is why Rosedale and I now believe protein restriction may be even more important than the restriction of net carbohydrates (total carbs minus fiber) from your diet.

This theory has in fact been tested and supported in mice, which admittedly are different from humans. The study was done in 2014 and published in *Cell Metabolism*;[6] longevity and health were boosted when carbohydrates replaced protein in the diets of mice, suggesting that reducing protein inhibits mTOR more than reducing carbs.

It's worth noting that the researchers didn't test a high-fat diet, and the study was done on mice, not humans. They were only looking at carbs versus protein, and if those were your only choices, protein restriction may in fact be more important than carb restriction. However, as I show throughout this book, there are many long-term drawbacks to eating excessive net carbs, so it seems a rational choice would be to replace net carbs with high-quality healthy *fats*, and restrict protein to just the amount your body needs for maintenance and repair.

It's also true that for young and maybe even midlife athletes, stimulating mTOR to build muscle and enjoy greater strength, speed, and performance is a worthy goal. It's important to remember that this is the group that is still capable of reproduction, and higher protein intake supports that as well. Most likely chronically suppressing mTOR, just like net carbs, is also an unwise strategy for optimizing health. I will discuss this in more depth in Chapter 10 on feast-and-famine cycling. Studies on this have yet to be done and no one knows for certain, but it seems prudent that once you pass your biological mandate to reproduce, you might be better served by focusing on how you can improve your health span and length of life by mostly suppressing mTOR with adequate protein levels, except on days when you are seeking to increase your muscle mass with strength training.

Another important exception would be those over 65 years old. The older you get the more important protein intake becomes to avoid lean muscle loss. So it would be wise to relax the restriction a bit in those who are older. Ideally larger intakes of protein would occur on days that strength training is used so the extra protein could be diverted to increased muscle.

An Interview with Dr. Ron Rosedale

In addition to Dr. Rosedale's work, Travis Christofferson, author of the excellent and must-read *Tripping over the Truth*, has also had a profound influence on me and inspired me to write this book. His writing style is so fluid and entertaining that I asked him to interview Dr. Rosedale for the book.

TC: Patients walking out of your clinic during the 1980s and '90s were often confused, because the things you typically told them ran against everything they had heard in the past. Regardless of their ailment—diabetes, cardiovascular disease, osteoporosis, cancer prevention, aches and pains, or simply trying to achieve better health—your prescription was the same: *eat fewer carbohydrates, less protein, and more fat.*

This was the pinnacle of the fat-phobic era. Your advice aggressively and directly challenged the prevailing dogma in a way that is unusual in the medical profession. I want to know more about how your thinking evolved over the years.

When did you first start to connect the dots that the medical community's thoughts on disease—and nutrition's role in it—were wrong?

RR: I started questioning conventional knowledge while I was still in medical school and we were learning about type 2 diabetes. I wondered, if a diabetic has high blood sugar, why would you feed him **more** sugar and then give him drugs to try and correct it? Yet that's what we were being taught—to treat blood sugar without addressing the real cause. The alternative seemed obvious: take away the carbohydrates that the body converts into sugar, and replace the calories with fat.

It seemed to me that simply managing symptoms was trying to pull a dandelion out by its leaves—you are not going to get very far. But the problem was, the medical establishment didn't know what the root was

When I was out of school and in my own practice, I put my patients on a low-carb, high-fat diet, and the results were remarkable.

One of my early cases was a man who showed up in my waiting room the day before he was scheduled for his second bypass surgery.

Without the surgery, he'd been told that he would be dead in a matter of weeks. He was willing to do anything to avoid another surgery, as his first bypass has been a horrific experience. He was in terrible shape. Every day he received 102 units of insulin, yet his blood sugar exceeded 300. Additionally, he was on eight different medications for other chronic medical conditions.

Instead of trying to treat each problem with drugs, I put him on a high-fat, low-carb diet and immediately took him off some medications while gradually weaning him off the rest.

I was aiming to restore cellular communication among the patient's 20 trillion cells until genes once again talked to genes and hormones talked to receptors40 The massive amounts of insulin flowing through the patient's veins were shouting instructions so loudly and abrasively that cells had quit listening, resulting in a problem known as insulin resistance. A reprieve from the constant shouting allowed cells to reestablish their insulin receptors so they could receive signals and then respond appropriately.

With communication restored between insulin and the rest of the body, many other problems began to resolve. Electrolyte balance was restored and blood vessels dilated, resulting in normal blood pressure. Vessel occlusions began to clear and nerves began to heal. The results were astonishing: no surgery, no more medications, no chest pain or neuropathy. This patient went on to play golf for 15 more years.

I treated many patients with different ailments the same way, and they experienced the same remarkable results.

The more conditions I treated with this type of diet, the more I saw that the multitude of chronic diseases afflicting society is deceptive. These diseases were just the symptoms—insulin was the root.

TC: You gave a landmark talk in 1999 called "Insulin and Its Metabolic Effects" that was widely reposted on the Internet and started to open some eyes and minds. Now in the 21st century, we know that insulin receptor resistance is a prime cause of mitochondrial dysfunction. What else helped you pull that together?

RR: In the 1980s and '90s, aging research was just cutting its teeth. I immersed myself in that research, driven by a hunch that the cause of many diseases arced back to the underappreciated process of aging—and I suspected insulin held the key.

Distilled to its essence, life has one imperative: to reproduce. Once our reproductive peak has passed, nature becomes apathetic to our survival, and we commence the process of programmed degeneration we call aging.

I learned that the corrosive effects of excess insulin can be observed outright. If you drip insulin into the femoral artery of a dog, as Dr. Anatolio B. Cruz, a surgeon and founding faculty member of University of Texas Health Science Center at San Antonio, accidentally noticed in the early '70s, the artery will become almost totally occluded with plaque in just over three months. It helped me see that insulin resistance was at the root of a myriad of corrosive aging processes, including elevated triglycerides, magnesium deficiencies, increasing cell division, the glycation of proteins, and the inhibition of autophagy (a process that rids the cell of debris).

In my mind, the answer appeared obvious: if the core of most people's medical problems stems from aging in general, and insulin and IGF-1 are signaling the body to age, then one should try to keep insulin and IGF-1 as low as possible, thus delaying aging while simultaneously switching on restorative pathways.

TC: As important as insulin is, you realized that leptin plays a role in obesity and chronic disease too. How did that come about?

RR: Leptin appeared to work through a straightforward mechanism—it determined a set point for fat accumulation. The set point is regulated by fat itself. In other words, fat determined its own fate by producing leptin.

I thought that once a person gained a healthy amount of fat, enough leptin was released into the bloodstream, where it traveled to the hypothalamus and gave specific instructions: stop eating and start burning fat. Conversely, if a person became too thin, the level of leptin would fall, signaling the body to eat more and store more fat. In essence, it seemed to me that leptin acted as a mediator of sorts, striking a balance between maintaining enough stored energy to survive a famine and preventing an organism from growing so large that it was unable to hunt or escape a predator.

But when researchers tested leptin levels in the obese, their levels were high, which contradicted everyone's understanding of how the hormone worked, including mine. I started to wonder if my anti-aging diet might work for leptin resistance as well. As with insulin, could it be as simple as removing the constant noise of too much leptin and allowing the hypothalamus and cells throughout the body time to "resensitize" themselves to leptin's signal?

Insulin and leptin receptor resistance are processes of desensitization, just as when you walk into a room with a strong smell, you eventually stop smelling it. You get resistant to the smell. But then when you leave the room for a while you get sensitized again, and when you go back in you can again detect the smell.

To test my theory, I needed a lab that could test for leptin. At the time, there was only one in the country that could do it. What I found was that by cutting out carbohydrates and certain amino acids (by reducing protein consumption), I would see patients' leptin levels drop by half in a few days. Not only were their leptin levels dropping, but also they weren't hungry and they were losing weight. They were reestablishing leptin sensitivity.

TC: What about the need to limit protein?

RR: The first piece I ascertained was that amino acids from protein could be converted into sugar, which in turn would stimulate insulin release. So although I knew protein was vital to health, I also started to see that there was a sweet spot of enough but not too much protein. Then I began to research mTOR, which is the master signaling pathway in the body to slow aging, and I saw that mTOR is powerfully influenced by protein consumption.

I felt that the other low-fat, high-carb diets advocated more protein than was healthy. I had seen in my own patients that if you restrict methionine, which is an amino acid that occurs in high levels in meat, you decrease visceral fat mass and you preserve insulin action, which decreases insulin, glucose, and leptin. You also get a gene expression profile that resembles one seen during treatment with rapamycin—one of the most powerful anticancer drugs known to man.

The Paleo diet tries to match diet to human evolution. But life has to strike a precarious balance between energy and reproduction, growth and repair, nurture and apathy. If you stimulate mTOR, your body will venture down the path toward aging and death—it's what it's programmed to do. What I'm trying to do with my diet is *unnatural*. I'm trying to intervene on nature itself to slow the aging process.

As we get older, excessive protein causes the cell to turn a blind eye to aging. But limiting it triggers a beautifully orchestrated network of internal processes that wards off disease, stretching out life and increasing the probability of exercising nature's imperative to reproduce. I put all this and more into a talk I gave in 2006 titled "Protein—the Good, the Bad, and the Ugly," which is available online if you type the title into a search engine.

The goal is to stretch out youth as long as possible, to avoid chronic disease, and to live a good life. All this is why I like to say, "Your health and life span are determined by the proportion of fat versus glucose you burn throughout your lifetime. And that is determined by what you choose to eat."

In many ways, health exists at the center of a teeter-totter. Eating protein can help you fuel muscular use, growth, and repair, but eating too much of it will lead to weight gain, aging, and disease. Nature gives with one hand while taking away with the other.

Fortunately, the key to slowing down the aging process is already in your hand—you simply need to stop eating more protein than your body requires for tissue repair. Reducing protein intake is so effective that it will likely become an even more visible component of anticancer and anti-aging dietary interventions in the future.

I'll cover how to determine exactly how much protein you need for your individual body to meet your needs without tipping the scale into excess in Chapter 8.

Using a High-Fat, Low-Carb Diet and Fasting Regime to Reverse Type 2 Diabetes

In October of 2015, Gino was diagnosed with type 2 diabetes. In an effort to better understand how his food choices affected his blood glucose, he began testing his fasting glucose levels before and after meals, late in the evening, and even in the middle of the night. He also adopted a low-glycemic diet designed specifically for people with diabetes, but saw only minimal improvement.

At his November visit to the diabetes clinic, the dietitian explained Canada's Food Guide, discussed the importance of exercise, and scheduled an appointment with Gino's primary care physician to get a prescription for Metformin, the drug so often prescribed to lower blood sugar in diabetic patients. Gino decided to follow the diet and exercise regimen but delay his primary care visit—he wanted to see what he could do on his own to improve his health without immediately turning to medication.

For the next few weeks, Gino followed the Food Guide recommendations. His daytime glucose readings were marginally lower, but both his fasting and his evening readings were exceptionally high. He couldn't understand how it was possible that his blood glucose levels were higher than before. (In fact, it was a textbook case of "dawn phenomenon," where people with diabetes experience a surge in glucose in the early-morning hours.)

By December Gino's efforts had yielded few results and he was discouraged because many of his glucose readings were higher than ever. In one last effort to avoid relying on medication to control his diabetes, he searched online for information regarding diabetes. That's how he found an online forum where people were discussing lifestyle changes that had reversed their diabetes and how he learned of Dr. Jason Fung, a nephrologist (kidney doctor) with extensive experience in using high-fat, low-carb diets in combination with different fasting regimens to treat patients with advanced diabetes.

Once Gino met with Dr. Fung, he adopted a low-carb, high-fat diet and scheduled his fasting periods to balance out the more carb-heavy traditional meals typically served at Christmas, New Year's, birthdays, and family dinners. He followed a 24-hour, alternate-day fasting schedule and created a system where any "indulgence" was quickly followed by a fast.

As of April 2016, just five months into the program, Gino's fasting glucose levels had returned to pre-diabetes levels and he'd lost 46 pounds. Now Gino reports that he actually looks forward to his fasts. "If I ever overindulge, I don't need to panic because I'm just one high-fat, low-carb meal and a short fast away from returning to normal levels. For me, this combination of leeway and control is the most amazing and motivating part of all."

CHAPTER 4

THE SURPRISING EFFECTS OF IRON ON MITOCHONDRIAL HEALTH

You likely think of iron as an important mineral that most people need to consume more of. But while it's true that having enough iron is an important factor of health, more is not better. In fact, high iron levels are serious threat to your health.

I know it can be difficult to reverse your thinking around a vital nutrient such as iron, especially if you have heard—either directly from your doctor or from the media—that you need to be sure you are getting plenty of it through your diet or supplements. But the research is clear: high iron levels can permanently damage your organs, tissues, and joints. Excess iron can also increase your risk of cancer, heart disease, and premature death; and that's just for starters.

There is a simple metabolic explanation for why this is so. It has to do with your mitochondria.

One of the normal products of mitochondrial respiration is hydrogen peroxide. Yes, the same one you can buy at the drugstore to clean infections. The hydrogen peroxide that is produced within your mitochondria as a normal part of ATP generation is healthy and necessary to regulate a variety of metabolic pathways. The problem occurs when your iron levels are too high. Through a process called the Fenton reaction, excess iron acts as a catalyst and transforms the relatively harmless hydrogen peroxide to hydroxyl free radical (OH^-). Without question, this is one of the most dangerous reactions that occur within your body because the hydroxyl free radical decimates mitochondrial DNA, proteins, and membranes. It also contributes to increased inflammation throughout your body, which is a precursor to all manner of chronic diseases.

This is why I suggest a blood test to determine your iron levels before embarking on MMT. You simply must have normal iron levels if you ever hope to optimize your mitochondrial function. You could be eating the perfect diet, but if your iron levels are high your mitochondrial health will suffer.

The good news is that iron overload is easy to treat—and easy to detect. All it requires is a simple blood test. In fact, I believe this is one of the most important tests that everyone should have done on a regular basis as part of a preventive, proactive health screening. But you need to know which test to get and not let physicians who are mostly uninformed about this danger lead you to get tests that will not accurately measure your risk of iron overload.

I'll discuss this in greater detail later in this chapter, but the test you want to get is a serum ferritin test. Ferritin is a protein within your cells that stores iron and releases it when your body needs it. It is a powerful predictor of the amount of stored iron in other locations and is the single most accurate and reliable indicator of iron overload.[1]

YOUR SEX AND YOUR AGE PLAY A LARGE ROLE IN YOUR IRON LEVELS

During their reproductive years, women shed 500 ml of iron each year through menstruation.[2] Indeed, the fact that women excrete iron each month for approximately 30 years is likely an important factor in why women have a longer life expectancy than men. Men don't have a method of regularly shedding significant amounts of iron, so their levels are consistently higher than premenopausal women.

Other than menstruation, the body has no natural mechanism for shedding any significant amount of iron. After menopause, women lose the benefit of shedding excess iron each month. Only about 1 milligram on average leaves the body through sweat, skin cell shedding, and very minor, normal bleeding in the GI tract, while the average amount of iron absorbed from nutritional intake is one to two milligrams.[3] This is why the older you are, the more important it is for you monitor and proactively reduce your iron levels.

In addition to damaging your mitochondria and contributing to genetic mutations, excess iron negatively impacts health in the following ways:

- **Promotion of growth of pathogens.** Iron facilitates growth. For this reason, it is essential for children to have enough iron in their bodies to sustain growth throughout childhood. Yet excessive iron in the body also facilitates growth of pathogenic bacteria, fungi, and protozoa[4] and makes your body a hospitable environment for microorganisms that can threaten your health.

- **Obesity.** The rise in supplemental iron intake over the last 70 years—beginning with the fortification of foods—correlates with rising obesity rates. Remember, iron is a growth factor. So just as low iron levels in pregnant women are associated with low birth weight babies, so are increased iron levels associated with weight gain.[5, 6] Studies have shown that obese people are likely to have elevated levels of ferritin.[7]

A large epidemiological study of adult men from Korea recently showed that moderately elevated levels of serum ferritin[8] predicted future weight gain, obesity, and even severe obesity. So if you picked up this book because you are struggling to lose the extra pounds you've gained, you have yet another reason to suspect that your failure to lose weight is not simply due to your diet or exercise regimen.

- **Diabetes.** Iron is believed to influence blood glucose and insulin levels,[9] and there is a correlation between serum ferritin levels and type 2 diabetes: In the Nurses' Health Study, which followed 30,000 disease-free men and women, elevated serum ferritin was associated with a significantly higher risk of type 2 diabetes.[10] Men with high iron stores were 2.4 times as likely to have type 2 diabetes as men with lower iron stores. Donating blood may also be beneficial in reducing your risk of developing diabetes, as frequent blood donors have been shown to have better insulin sensitivity and a decreased risk of diabetes.[11]

- **Cardiovascular disease.** The same Nurses' Health Study also found that those who had donated blood were 50 percent less likely to have a stroke or heart attack. Iron likely plays a role in heart disease by participating in the oxidation of LDL and damage of endothelial cells, both of which contribute to athero-sclerosis.[12, 13]

  Since the 1980s, researchers have hypothesized that gender differences in iron levels could explain the higher prevalence of heart disease in men. Patholo-gist Dr. Jerome Sullivan first posited the theory in a paper published in *The Lancet* titled "Iron and the Sex Difference in Heart Disease Risk." The Nurses' Health Study found that women's risk of heart disease rose significantly after they either went through menopause naturally or had a hysterectomy—in other words, when they stopped excreting iron through menstruation each month—suggesting that there is a link between iron levels and cardiovascular disease.[14]

- **Neurodegenerative diseases, including Alzheimer's disease, Parkinson's disease, and ALS.** The brain has a larger requirement for oxygen than any other organ, and iron is essential to delivering oxygen where it is needed. But like everywhere else in the body, excess iron in the brain is decidedly not a good thing. Indeed, the fact that levels of iron increase as we get older likely explains, at least in part, why neurodegenerative diseases such as Alzheimer's disease and Parkinson's disease are associated with aging. Iron is found in high concentrations in the plaques found in the brains of Alzheimer's patients[15] and in abnormal concentrations in the brains of patients with early-onset Alzheimer's disease and Parkinson's disease.[16, 17]

    A 2014 study found that elevated ferritin levels in cerebrospinal fluid predicted the conversion of mild cognitive impairment to full-blown Alzheimer's disease.[18] Higher levels of iron in the brain have also been shown to correlate with the severity of cognitive impairment.[19] Oxidative stress and the resulting inflammation are likely the mechanisms involved in how excess iron impairs brain function.

- **Cancer.** Excess iron contributes to cancer by damaging your mitochondrial DNA through excessive hydroxyl free radical generation. Serum ferritin is elevated in patients with many types of cancers, including pancreatic cancer, breast cancer, melanoma, renal cell carcinoma, and Hodgkin's lymphoma.[20] Analysis of the National Health and Nutrition Examination Survey showed a link between dietary intake and body iron stores and the risk of colorectal cancer.

Body iron stores are also positively associated with polyps and precancerous lesions in the colon. Iron may be why consumption of red meat is a risk factor for colon cancer, as excess iron could promote inflammation in the colon that leads to mucosal damage. Dietary fiber is thought to help prevent this, since fiber binds to iron and helps the metal pass out of the body through the digestive tract.[21] Similar data exist to support the belief that iron excess contributes to liver cancer.[22] Providing further evidence of the link between excess iron and cancer, those who regularly donate blood have a lower risk of cancer. A randomized trial found that blood draws reduced incidence of all cancers by 37 percent.[23]

- **Osteoporosis.** Sufficient iron levels are important to maintain your bone health, which is regulated by cells that are iron sensitive. Simply put, excessive iron will damage your bones. This explains why people with iron-loading disorders, such as hemochromatosis, are more likely to have osteoporosis.[24]

How Do You Know if You Have Excess Iron?

Because the dangers of excess iron are so great, and because symptoms associated with this excess don't typically appear until iron levels are already dangerously high, it is important to have your blood tested regularly to help gauge your risk. And given that your health care providers may not understand what your lab results mean, you may need to look beyond your current team to find someone who is more knowledgeable in this area (I provide more information on how to get this test in Chapter 6).

Symptoms of Excess Iron

Unfortunately, iron levels sufficient to harm your health do not cause any immediate symptoms (just like high blood pressure or vitamin D deficiency). If they remain severely elevated for prolonged periods, however, they can cause the following symptoms:[25, 26]

- Joint pain
- Bronze or gray color to your skin, also known as "bronze diabetes"
- Irregular heartbeat
- Fatigue
- Abdominal pain
- Heart flutters
- Memory fog

The Importance of Accurate Testing

As is shown in the table below, physicians use several tests to check iron status. The problem is that most physicians have not carefully studied this area and therefore do not appreciate the importance of the most important screening test to measure ferritin levels in your body. Many will perform the other tests and falsely reassure you that your iron levels are normal and you have nothing to worry about.

Test	Reference Range[27]
Serum ferritin	Men: 20–200 ng/mL (nanogram per milliliter) Women: 15–150 ng/mL
Serum iron	60–170 mcg/dL (micrograms per deciliter)
Total iron binding capacity	240– 450 mcg/dL
Transferrin saturation	20–50 percent

The most important test, serum ferritin, measures the amount of ferritin in your blood. The next two lab tests are used to calculate the transferrin saturation: serum iron, which measures the amount of circulating iron, and total iron binding capacity, which measures the ability of the transferrin molecule to carry iron.[28]

Please understand that the recommendation is for a serum ferritin test and not a serum iron or total iron binding capacity test, both of which can be normal even though the ferritin is elevated. So don't let your doctor talk you out of getting this test for one they feel is better. It isn't.

As you can see, there is a fairly wide window of acceptable levels, but the ranges currently viewed as "healthy" do not reflect optimal levels. This is similar to how we once viewed vitamin D levels: for much of the 20th century, only levels under 20 ng/mL of vitamin D were thought to be deficient, but more recent science has shown that you need at least 40 ng/mL to be in a healthy range.

The disparity between acceptable and optimal reference ranges for ferritin is even worse. To put a finer point on it, multiple epidemiological studies have linked increased longevity with serum ferritin levels below a threshold of 80–90 ng/mL, which is a typical plateau for postmenopausal women.[29] The healthy range of serum ferritin lies between 20 and 80 ng/mL. Below 20, you are iron deficient, and above 80, you have an iron surplus. Women in their reproductive years have an average ferritin level of 35 ng/mL, while men in the same age range have an average level of 150 ng/mL.[30] Ferritin levels can go really high. I've seen levels over 1,000, but anything over 80 is likely going to be a problem. The ideal range is 40–60 ng/mL.

TESTING MY DAD'S IRON LEVELS SAVED HIS LIFE

I first became aware of the dangers of excess iron about 20 years ago. At that time, I checked my dad's ferritin level and was shocked to discover that it was close to 1,000. While some of that was likely due to his age (65), most of the excess was a result of beta thalassemia, a hereditary blood disorder that causes a high turnover of red blood cells and leads to an accumulation of iron.

With regular blood draws, his iron levels normalized, but the high iron levels had already damaged his pancreatic islet cells. Now he has what is called "bronze" diabetes that requires him to use insulin. Without early detection of this disease, I am absolutely sure he would have died 10 or 15 years ago. As I write this now as he is approaching 90 years old.

I inherited beta thalassemia from him. Fortunately, I learned while I was still young and unaffected by it that I needed to carefully control my iron levels and in doing so have managed to sidestep the problems associated with this genetic disease. I aim to keep my serum ferritin under 60 ng/mL by removing about 4 ounces of blood every six weeks.

How to Keep Your Iron Levels in Check

There is no magic supplement to take to remove iron from your body. The safest, most effective, and typically least expensive way to remove excess iron is simply to remove blood from your body since your red blood cells are loaded with hemoglobin that contain large stores of iron.

If you determine that you have excess iron levels, you'll want to schedule blood donations to lower serum ferritin. Blood donation is a simple and life-giving way to treat iron overload while helping others at the same time. One blood donation reduces ferritin by somewhere between 30 and 50 ng/mL.[31] Here are my recommendations for your blood donation schedule:

Ferritin Level	Donation schedule
< 60 ng/mL	Donation not necessary
100–125 ng/mL	Donate 1 to 2 times yearly
126–200 ng/mL	Donate 2 to 3 times yearly
201–250 ng/mL	Donate 3 to 4 times yearly
>250 ng/mL	Donate every two months if possible

If for any reason you are unwilling or unable to obtain the ferritin test, you may want to consider a general recommendation based on average levels for your age and gender. If you are a postmenopausal female or adult male, you should ideally donate blood two or three times a year to minimize your iron stores. If you are still menstruating, it would be best to have your ferritin level tested and follow the table above.

If you are unable to donate your blood due to age, low weight, or other contraindications, you can get a prescription for therapeutic phlebotomy, which is a fancy word for taking your blood in order to treat a condition. Most any center that accepts blood donations is now required by federal law to accept your prescription for a therapeutic phlebotomy. (The blood is disposed of, not used.)

Alternatively, the best and most convenient option is what I do: find someone you know who can draw blood and come to your home to remove 2 to 4 ounces of blood every month. This creates far less metabolic stress on your biology and closely resembles the iron loss that happens in a woman's natural menstrual cycle.

Additionally, you should make sure that you aren't consuming unhealthful levels of iron, nor absorbing too much of the iron you end up consuming. You can do this in two ways:

1. Minimize factors that increase iron absorption, including:

   - Cooking in iron pots or pans, as these vessels leach some of their iron into the foods you prepare in them. Cooking acidic foods—such as tomato sauce—in iron pots or pans will cause even more iron to leach into your foods.

- Eating processed food products like cereals and white breads that are "fortified" with iron. The iron they use in these products is a low-quality inorganic iron, similar to rust, and it is far more dangerous than the natural heme iron (which means "blood iron") found in meat.

- Drinking well water that is high in iron. The key to minimizing the iron levels in your drinking water is to make sure you have some type of iron precipitator and/or a reverse osmosis water filter.

- Taking multiple vitamins and mineral supplements that have iron in them. Check your supplements carefully.

- Taking vitamin C supplements or fortified juices with meals, as it increases absorption. Even something as simple as eating tomatoes with beef will increase absorption.

- Overconsuming animal protein. As I discussed in Chapter 3, most Americans eat way too much protein in general—more than the body truly needs, with the excess getting converted into glucose and stored as fat. The other peril of eating too much meat is that it contains a lot of heme iron. While it is less dangerous than the inorganic forms of iron found in fortified foods, your body has no mechanism to stop absorption of heme iron when there is already plenty on hand, so please let this information help you stick to your protein intake target (calculated as 1 gram per kilogram of lean body mass).

- Drinking alcohol, as it increases the absorption of any iron in your diet. For instance, if you drink a martini with your steak, you will likely be absorbing more iron than is healthy for you.

2. Decrease iron absorption—carefully—in the following ways:

   - Drink black tea, which inhibits iron absorption by up to 95 percent (the same cannot be said for green, white, or herbal teas).

   - Take calcium, as calcium inhibits iron absorption. If you take any supplemental calcium, it is best to consume it with the meal that has the most iron in it.

   - Drink red wine, which inhibits absorption of about 65 percent of the iron in foods.

   - Drink coffee, which has an effect similar to black tea, with a strong impact on inhibiting absorption of iron from food.[32]

   - Go for periods without consuming food, as in my recommended Peak Fasting (see page 224 for more information). This increases hepcidin, a hormone that reduces the absorption of iron from food.[33]

   - Exercise regularly, as it changes the way your body absorbs iron by lowering overall uptake, which may explain why athletes are more prone to iron deficiency.[34]

A final strategy you may wish to pursue, particularly if blood draws are unavailable or seem too extreme to you, is to take low-dose aspirin. Aspirin has long been associated with a decreased risk of heart disease. It was thought this effect was due to its influence on thinning your blood, but it is more likely due to the fact that iron causes low-level, often undetectable, bleeding in the intestines, and over time it lowers iron levels. Taking an aspirin every day results in essentially the same iron level reduction as giving blood, although it can take years of regular use to achieve the same therapeutic benefits as phlebotomies. This reduction in iron levels may be the reason numerous studies have found that long-term use of low-dose aspirin has major anticancer benefits, including 75 percent lower rates of esophageal cancer, 20 percent lower overall cancer rate, and 50 percent lower risk of metastasis.[35]

CHAPTER 5

WHAT TO EAT ON MMT: THE CLEANEST, MOST EFFICIENT FUEL FOR YOUR BODY

As I covered in Chapter 1, one of the greatest powers of MMT is that you can use it to avoid overproduction of ROS in your cells. MMT achieves this balance in three primary ways: the food you eat (which I'll outline in just a moment), when you eat it (which I will cover in Chapter 10), and keeping tabs on your iron levels (which I covered in Chapter 4).

In this chapter I'll discuss the three major categories of foods—carbs, protein, and fats—called "macronutrients" and provide examples of specific foods that work best on MMT within each of category.

Use this chapter to start reorienting your thinking on what to eat and to make grocery lists. You can begin incorporating more of these foods now, even before you've officially started MMT, thereby giving your palate some time to adjust. Although all the foods on this list are delicious in themselves and when used in recipes, it can be a process to wean yourself off processed foods and high-carb staples such as bread and pasta. Let this chapter inspire you to start making different food choices right away.

CARBOHYDRATES

The most efficient way to train your body to use fat for fuel and reduce your exposure to free radical damage is to limit the number of net carbs you get from your diet.

Limiting net carbs is a crucial part of MMT not just because glucose is a "dirty" fuel that produces an excess of ROS, but also because excessive net carbohydrate consumption suppresses fat burning. Notice that I say "net carbs": that's total carbs minus fiber. Thus MMT is not a low-*total*-carb diet—because fiber is an important carb that actually converts to beneficial short-chain fats in your intestine. Rather, this is a low-*net*-carb diet.

If you look at the nutrition facts label on a processed food package, it will list total carbs—that figure is not what I'm talking about. You need to also look at the fiber content and subtract that from the total carbs. This is important to understand, or else you may end up feeling that your choices are too limited to keep to your MMT food plan.

By dramatically reducing the number of net-fiber carbs that you eat, you will need to fill the calorie void with other types of foods. On MMT, you will replace those nonfiber carb calories (from foods such as sweets, sugary beverages, breads, pasta, crackers, chips, and fries) with organic vegetables and healthy fats. This will transition your body into primarily burning fat for fuel while radically reducing your risk for most chronic diseases.

In general, the high volume of vegetables, together with the nuts and seeds you eat while following MMT (which I'll cover just a few pages from now), will provide you with more daily fiber than the average American typically eats.

The vegetables you want to prioritize are the low-carb kinds. Think celery, greens, and cauliflower (relatively few carbs) versus carrots, sweet potatoes, and potatoes (relatively high carbs). Although sweet potatoes, for example, are whole foods and have many nutritional benefits in terms of vitamins and minerals, they are simply too high in carbohydrates—which, remember, your body converts into glucose—to comply with MMT. Particularly when you start on the program, the number of carbs in a sweet potato can prevent you from making the shift to fat burning.

The same is true for fruit, which typically contains natural sugars that are then converted to glucose once you eat them. (However, there are a handful of fruits that have low levels of naturally occurring sugars, which you can eat in small amounts with careful monitoring—I cover those in just a moment.) The less fruit you eat, particularly when you first start following MMT, the easier it will be for you to transition to burning fat.

Here are the veggies and fruits that are part of MMT.

MMT-Friendly Vegetables

- Asparagus
- Avocados
- Broccoli
- Brussels sprouts
- Cabbage
- Cauliflower
- Celery
- Cucumbers
- Kale
- Mushrooms
- Salad greens
- Sauté greens

- Spinach
- Zucchini

After you are fat adapted, you can add back limited amounts of these foods:

- Eggplant
- Garlic
- Onions
- Parsnips
- Peppers
- Rutabaga
- Tomatoes
- Winter squash (very limited amounts)

MMT-Friendly Fruits

- Berries (a small handful, in lieu of a serving of vegetables)
- Grapefruit (a few sections, also instead of a serving of vegetables)

The reason these vegetables and fruits make the list is that they are low in carbs and high in fiber. However, fiber is such an important component of health that I recommend you go beyond food sources and take it as a supplement.

Fiber is a crucial component of MMT for four primary reasons:

- Fiber is used as food for your beneficial bacteria, and a healthy microbiome is essential to optimizing your health. (For a deeper dive into how and why to nurture your gut microbiome, refer to my previous book *Effortless Healing*.)

- The insoluble fiber you consume is passed through your body undigested while the soluble fiber is converted to short-chain fatty acids that nourish your healthy gut bacteria, are used as fuel by your cells, and serve as important biological signaling molecules.

- Fiber acts as an antinutrient—it reduces absorption of carbohydrates, meaning it reduces glucose and insulin peaks.[1]

- Insoluble fiber also forms a latticework in your intestine, and the soluble fiber plugs the holes. Together they form a barrier that helps protect your liver.

I've been interested in the health benefits of fiber for a long time—so much so that my classmates nicknamed me "Dr. Fiber" when I was in medical school in the '70s. Today, I still hold firm to my belief in the benefits of dietary fiber as long as most of it is coming from high-quality (preferably organic) vegetables and low-net-carb grains. (Fortunately, I lost the nickname Dr. Fiber.)

Fiber undoubtedly contributes to overall good health and longevity, and can have a positive impact on lowering your risk of disease by feeding and promoting the proliferation of healthy gut bacteria. In recent years it's become crystal clear that in order to be truly healthy, you need a healthy gut.

When your beneficial gut bacteria are fueled by plenty of fiber, they produce compounds that help regulate your immune function and even improve brain health. For starters, these compounds help increase the number of regulatory T cells—specialized immune system cells that help prevent autoimmune responses and more. Regulatory T cells are also involved in the formation of other specialized blood cells in your body via a process called hematopoiesis.

When fiber is lacking, these beneficial bacteria starve, which can send your health into a downward spiral. This has a negative impact not only on your immune system and the development of autoimmune diseases, but also in your gut. There, it causes the breakdown of the protective gut barrier, which can lead to leaky gut syndrome. People with this disorder often suffer from widespread inflammation and inflammatory diseases.

Researchers have also found that a diet high in fiber is associated with a lower risk of premature death from *any* cause, likely because it helps reduce your risk of a number of life-threatening chronic diseases, including type 2 diabetes, heart disease, stroke, and cancer.

Studies have also linked a high-fiber diet to beneficial reductions in cholesterol and blood pressure, improved insulin sensitivity, and reduced inflammation—all of which can influence your mortality risk. There are two types of fiber:

- **Soluble fiber,** like that found in cucumbers, berries, beans, and nuts, forms a gel-like mass in the gut, helping *slow down* your digestion. This leaves you feeling fuller for a longer period of time and is one reason why fiber may help with fat loss. It also slows glucose uptake, resulting in lower net insulin levels. This type of fiber ferments in the gut and is responsible for maintaining the health of your microbiome.

- **Insoluble fiber,** found in foods like dark-green leafy vegetables, green beans, and celery, does not break down during digestion. It has many benefits, and two of the most important are its ability to bind to toxins, aiding in their elimination, and its ability to stabilize the pH in your intestines, creating an inhospitable environment for potentially harmful microbes. Insoluble fiber helps speed the transit of waste products, helping you maintain regular bowel movements. It is also a powerful stool normalizer, and if you are constipated it will soften your stools by drawing water into the colon, which adds bulk. If you have loose stools it will make them more solid by absorbing excess water. Insoluble fiber also scrubs the lining of your colon. There's a sweet spot here: enough scrubbing to remove toxins and waste but not so much that you're scrubbing away the protective mucosal lining. Another fact to note is that this type of fiber can bind to and remove minerals and medications, so if you're taking a fiber supplement, timing is important. It's best to allow an hour or so on either side of taking a soluble fiber supplement.

Many whole foods, especially vegetables, fruits, nuts, and seeds, naturally contain *both* soluble and insoluble fiber. I recommend consuming a minimum of 35 grams of fiber and ideally 50 grams or more from whole foods a day, but you could easily double or even triple that amount. My personal consumption is about two and half times that, 75 grams per day.

If you fall short of the recommended 35 grams, or meet that total but want to consume greater amounts so you can experience more of its benefits, I recommend supplementing with organic psyllium seeds (there is more information about how to do this in Appendix B). This is a relatively inexpensive and easy way to add more soluble fiber. I personally take one tablespoon three times a day. Just make sure that the psyllium is organic. Avoid nonorganic psyllium like the plague as it is loaded with pesticides. Taking organic psyllium powder is also helpful in counteracting the loose stools that many experience when taking MCT oil (which I cover in the next section). For additional fiber I also take two to three tablespoons of chia seeds daily. Additionally I soak one tablespoon of flax seeds overnight and blend those into my smoothie. It is important to note that if your gut is not used to these amounts of fiber, you will want to gradually increase to those levels, as they can cause gas and bloating and even constipation until your microbiome readjusts.

THREE OF THE SAFEST SUGAR ALTERNATIVES

Turning down the volume on your sweet tooth and avoiding nearly all sugars—natural and artificial—is a crucial piece of your success on MMT. I know how daunting a task like this can be. But there's good news: Once you have made the switch to fat burning, your cravings for sugar will almost magically disappear. You will no longer feel that "need" for dessert after every meal, nor will you be driven to have a sugary snack in the mid-afternoon to ward off an energy crash.

1. **Sugar alcohols** have "ol" at the end of their name—these include erythritol, xylitol, sorbitol, maltitol, mannitol, and glycerol. They're not as sweet as sugar, and they do contain fewer calories, but they're not calorie free. So don't get confused by the "sugar free" label on foods containing these sweeteners. As with all foods, you need to carefully read the food labels for calorie and carbohydrate content, regardless of any claims that the food is sugar free or low sugar.

   Erythritol is by far the darling of the keto world, replacing xylitol in most recipes. It's the most tolerable and, unlike xylitol, there's no fermentation in the gut and I haven't seen any evidence—yet—of disruption in the microbiome. However, I strongly suggest that you limit its use so you do not become dependent on it.

   One reason sugar alcohols provide fewer calories than sugar is that they're not completely absorbed into your body. Instead, most sugar alcohols are fermented in the gut. Because of this, eating too many foods containing sugar alcohols can lead to abdominal gas and diarrhea. It's also worth noting that maltitol, a commonly used sugar alcohol, spikes blood sugar almost as much as a high-net-carb new potato. Xylitol and erythritol, in comparison, do not have a great effect on your blood sugar, so from that perspective may be a better choice in small quantities if you feel the need to sweeten.

   In summary, some sugar alcohols are a far superior alternative to highly refined sugar, fructose, or artificial sweeteners if they are consumed in moderation. Of the various sugar alcohols, xylitol and erythritol are two of the best. In their pure state, the potential side effects are minimal, and xylitol actually comes with some benefits such as fighting tooth decay. All in all, I would say that xylitol is reasonably safe, and potentially even a mildly beneficial sweetener. (As a side note, xylitol is toxic to dogs and some other animals, so be sure to keep it out of reach of your family pets.)

2. **Stevia** is a highly sweet herb derived from the leaf of the South American stevia plant. It is sold as a liquid and as a powder and is completely safe in its natural form. It can be used to sweeten most dishes and drinks, although be careful with it—because it's so sweet, a little goes a long way. Keep in mind that the same cannot be said for Truvia, which makes use of only certain active ingredients of stevia and not the entire plant. Usually it's the *synergistic* effect of all the agents in the plant that provides the overall health effect, which oftentimes includes "built-in protection" against potentially damaging effects. Truvia *may* turn out to be a very good substitute to sugar, but I'd have to see more details before giving it an enthusiastic thumbs-up, as there's just not enough evidence to prove its safety.

3. **Lo han kuo** is another natural sweetener similar to stevia, but it's a bit more expensive and harder to find. In China, the lo han fruit has been used as a sweetener for centuries, and it's about 200 times sweeter than sugar. It received FDA GRAS (generally regarded as safe) status in 2009.

FATS

There are no two ways about it: MMT is a high-fat diet. To promote your shift to fat burning, you want to get the majority of your calories from fat. But you must choose your fats wisely.

It's imperative that you choose healthy fats (which I'll go over in just a moment) and eliminate *all* industrially processed fats—including vegetable oils such as canola, peanut, cottonseed, corn, and soy—as well as all trans fats, such as those found in commercial salad dressings, peanut butter, most mayonnaise, and anything processed or packaged. It's important that you read the ingredients, not just the label: if you see "hydrogenated fat" listed in the ingredients, that food contains trans fats, even if they're at a level below what needs to be reported on the label.

As I covered in detail in Chapter 1, refined oils are deadly for a wide variety of reasons: they throw your omega-6 to omega-3 ratio out of balance, they are highly susceptible to oxidation (which kicks off a storm of free radical damage within your mitochondria), they carry high levels of pesticides because most vegetable oils are extracted from genetically modified glyphosate-soaked plants, and they become even more volatile and harmful when they are subjected to heat.

If you decide to personally adopt MMT, which I sincerely hope you will do, but you replace your current high-carb calories with calories from industrially processed fats, you will not enjoy any benefits from this diet. Instead, you'll be creating even more harm to your mitochondria and overall health.

Here are the sources of fat that burn clean and help heal your mitochondria (and since many sources of high-quality fats also come packaged with protein, there are several more—such as grass-fed beef and pastured eggs—listed in the protein section).

- Organic, grass-fed butter and ghee
- Coconut milk
- Chicken fat
- Duck fat
- Coconut oil
- MCT oil
- Avocado oil
- Extra virgin olive oil

Coconut and MCT Oil

Coconut oil has been a dietary and beauty staple for millennia. It fights all kinds of microbes, from viruses to bacteria to protozoa, many of which can be harmful, and is a fabulous source of high-quality fat.

Around 50 percent of the fat in coconut oil is lauric acid, which is rarely found in nature. In fact, coconut oil has a greater proportion of lauric acid than any other food. Your body converts lauric acid into monolaurin, a monoglyceride (a single fat attached to a glycerol molecule, unlike three fats which would be a triglyceride) that can actually destroy many lipid-coated viruses such as HIV, herpes, influenza, measles, gram-negative bacteria, and protozoa such as *Giardia lamblia*.

For a quick hunger buster or energy boost, you could simply eat a spoonful of coconut oil. You can also add coconut oil to your tea or coffee in lieu of a sweetener. Coconut also helps improve absorption of fat-soluble vitamins, so taking a spoonful of coconut oil along with your daily vitamins may help boost their effectiveness.

If you want to heighten the benefits of MMT, I also recommend adding MCT oil to your daily plan.

MCT oil is coconut oil's more concentrated cousin. Derived from coconut oil, most commercially-available MCT consists of equal amounts of caprylic acid (C8, a fatty acid with 8 carbon atoms in its molecular structure) and capric acid (C10, a 10-carbon fatty acid).

Normally, when you eat a fatty food, it is broken down in the small intestine primarily through the action of bile salts and lipase, a pancreatic enzyme. But medium-chain triglycerides are able to bypass this process; they diffuse across the intestinal membrane and go directly to your liver via the hepatic portal. Once there, especially if you are in nutritional ketosis, or burning fat for fuel, they are quickly converted into ketones, which are then released back into your bloodstream and are transported throughout your body, including to your brain, to be used as a clean-burning fuel.

For this reason, MCT oil is a great way to take in some extra fat, as it is odorless and tasteless and is therefore easy to consume straight off the spoon. Its rapid conversion to energy can help you stay on the MMT plan in those moments where your hunger is high and appropriate food is scarce.

The only hitch is that this efficiency does come with a small cost. Your liver may not be able to process that much fat quickly, and so may dump some of it back into your intestines, where it can cause stomach upset and loose stools. You can consume MCT oil every day, but you must start slowly and build up your dosage over time so you can increase your tolerance to it. (For this reason, MCT oil can help also ease constipation, but don't overdo it just to get that effect.)

Start with one teaspoon once a day, preferably combined with food, and if you don't experience loose stools or other GI symptoms, gradually work your way up. Some people use up to a tablespoon or two with each meal, but most only need a tablespoon or two per day. If at any point you develop digestive upset, go back to your previous dose and stay there for a few days. Increasing your fiber intake can also help ward off MCT oil–induced diarrhea and bloating. Aim to eat approximately 25 grams of fiber for every tablespoon of MCT oil.

My personal preference, even though it is more expensive, is straight C8 (caprylic acid), as it converts to ketones far more rapidly and efficiently than do the other versions of MCT oil, most of which contain close to a 50:50 combination of C8 and C10 (capric acid) fats. It may be easier on your digestion as well. Whatever MCT oil you buy, be sure to store it away from sunlight in an opaque bottle that limits light exposure.

Although MCT is not usually used as a cooking oil, you can still use it in some recipes; just avoid heating it over 320 degrees. For example, you can substitute it for part of the oil that you would use to make mayonnaise or a salad dressing, blend it with vegetables to make a sauce, or add it to smoothies or soups. You can also add it to coffee or tea along with another fat like ghee; blend it well and enjoy it for an energy boost.

There's just one thing to keep in mind: because MCT oil is so readily converted to fuel, and that fuel can be utilized by your brain and heart, if you take it at night you may be too hyperalert to sleep. That said, if you are following the whole MMT program, you will be avoiding all food for a minimum of three hours before sleep (as I will outline in Chapter 10), so this effect should not be an issue.

Caution: Individuals with liver cancer, elevated liver enzymes, extensive liver metastases, or liver disease *should not* use MCT oil. However, they can still use coconut oil.

Avocados

Avocados are one of the healthiest foods you can eat. Personally, I eat one to three almost every day. They are an excellent source of healthy monounsaturated fat—a type your body can easily burn for energy—and vitamins and antioxidants. These super fruits have numerous other benefits:

- **Weight loss.** According to research published in
  Nutrition Journal, those who ate half an avocado with
  their standard lunch reported being 40 percent less
  hungry three hours after their meal and 28 percent
  less hungry at the five-hour mark compared to those
  who did not eat avocado with lunch. The study also
  found that avocados appear helpful for regulating
  blood sugar.[2]

- **Nutrient rich.** Avocados provide close to 20 essential
  health-boosting nutrients, including potassium, vitamin E, B vitamins, and folic acid. Potassium plays
  an important role in heart function, skeletal health,
  digestion, and muscular function, and is essential for
  the proper function of all cells, tissues, and organs in
  your body.[3] Despite the fact that it is available in many
  foods, only 2 percent of U.S. adults get the recommended daily amount.[4] This is particularly troubling

because potassium offsets the hypertensive effects of sodium. Imbalance in your sodium-potassium ratio can not only lead to high blood pressure, but may also contribute to a number of *other* diseases, including heart disease and stroke.

About two and a half avocados provide the daily recommended amount of about 4,700 milligrams (mg) of potassium a day. Additionally, an average avocado contains about 40 mg of magnesium, which is about 10 percent of the recommended daily value.

Magnesium is another mineral that is important to balance with calcium. By some estimates, up to 80 percent of Americans are not getting enough magnesium and may be deficient. If you suffer from unexplained fatigue or weakness, abnormal heart rhythms, or even muscle spasms and eye twitches, low levels of magnesium could be to blame.

Better still, avocados are one of few foods that contain significant levels of both vitamins C and E[5] and are high in fiber, with about 4.6 grams in half an avocado. So when you eat avocados, you're really providing your body with a comprehensive package of nutrition.

- **Nutrient absorption boosting.** Because they are so rich in healthy fats, avocados help your body absorb fat-soluble nutrients from other foods. One study published in *The Journal of Nutrition* found that consuming a whole fresh avocado with either an orange-colored tomato sauce or raw carrots significantly enhanced absorption of the carotenoids and conversion of them into an active form of vitamin A.[6] A 2005 study similarly found that adding avocado to salad allowed the volunteers to absorb *three to five times* more carotenoid antioxidant molecules, which help protect your body against free radical damage.[7]

- **Cancer fighting.** Avocatin B, a type of fat found in avocados, has been found to combat acute myeloid leukemia, which is a particularly rare and deadly form of cancer. The avocado fat was able to wipe out the leukemia stem cells while leaving healthy cells unharmed.[8] Avocados are also rich in cancer-fighting carotenoids, which are most plentiful in the dark-green portion of the flesh that's closest to the skin.

I even take avocados with me when I travel, making sure to take really hard ones, as they will ripen perfectly during the trip without getting crushed in my bag. You can use any type of rigid container, but I like to transport them in a rigid cardboard tube to prevent them from being squashed in my checked luggage.

Avocados have been rated as one of the safest commercial crops in terms of pesticide application, and their thick skin protects the inner fruit from pesticides. So there's no real need to spend extra money on organic avocados. I've even had my own team test avocados from a variety of growers in different countries, sold in several major grocery stores, and they all tested free and clear of harmful chemicals.

To preserve the area with the greatest concentration of antioxidants, you basically want to peel the avocado with your hands, as you would a banana:

- First, cut the avocado lengthwise, around the seed
- Holding each half, twist them in opposite directions to separate them from the seed
- Remove the seed
- Cut each half, lengthwise
- Next, using a teaspoon or your thumb and index finger, simply peel the skin off each piece

One note: If you have a latex allergy, you may have a cross-reaction to avocados. Also, if you suffer from seasonal allergies, you may notice a sensitivity to avocados when the pollen count is high. You may want to take periodic breaks from daily avocado consumption so you don't develop an allergy or sensitivity to them.

Despite all these benefits, avocados do have one serious drawback: They can be expensive, particularly if you don't live in a state where they are grown. To offset some of their cost, purchase them when they are on sale—choose ones that are green and rock hard. You can keep them in the fridge for up to three weeks; simply take them out two days before you want to eat them to allow them to ripen and soften.

Olives and Olive Oil

Olives are a wonder of nature that are easy to take for granted, yet deserve special attention. One hundred grams (3.5 ounces) of olive oil has nearly 100 grams of fat: monounsaturated (77 grams), polyunsaturated (8.4 grams), and saturated (13.5 grams). Olives are a great, satiating snack, salty and satisfying, and a wonderful addition to salads. They are a healthful way to add more fat to your diet. Olives, olive oil, and the compounds they contain have been linked to the following health benefits:

- **Antioxidant powerhouse.** Olives contain high quantities of several different antioxidants, including phenols (hydroxytyrosol, tyrosol), polyphenols (oleuropein glucoside), and oleuropein, which is only found in olives. The antioxidant properties of olives have been shown to be stronger than those of vitamin E.

- **Heart protection.** Most of the fat in olives and olive oil is oleic acid, a monounsaturated fat known for lowering your risk of heart disease by decreasing LDL cholesterol and blood pressure. Oleuropein, an antioxidant component of olives, also reduces the oxidation of LDL cholesterol in your body and may lower markers of oxidative stress.

- **Anticancer activity.** The antioxidant and anti-inflammatory properties in olives, as well as other anticancer compounds, make them useful for cancer prevention. For instance, compounds in olives and olive oil have been found to activate the tumor suppressor gene and apoptotic gene, which induces programmed cell death.[9]

- **Anti-aging benefits.** Tyrosol, a phenol found in extra virgin olive oil, has been found to increase life span and resistance to stress in roundworms.[10] Oleuropein, hydroxytyrosol (another antioxidant), and squalene in olives may also help protect your skin against the radiation in ultraviolet (UV) light; oleuropein in particular has been found to act as a skin protector and has direct antioxidant action on your skin.[11]

- **Bone health.** Consumption of olive oil and olives has been shown to prevent the loss of bone mass in animal studies of age-related osteoporosis. In a study of 127 elderly men, consumption of a Mediterranean diet enriched with virgin olive oil for two years was associated with increased bone-building proteins, which suggests olives may have protective effects on bone.[12] Phenolic compounds in extra virgin olive oil have also been found to stimulate human osteoblastic cell proliferation[13] (osteoblasts are bone-forming cells).

It's relatively easy to find high-quality olives (look for those with the pits intact and sold in a jar, not a can), but this isn't the case for olive oil. According to the U.S. Pharmacopeial Convention's Food Fraud Database,[14] olive oil is commonly and deliberately diluted with less expensive and inferior quality oils, including hazelnut, soybean, corn, sunflower, palm, sesame, grape seed, and frequently inferior, non-human-grade olive oils, as they more easily evade fraud detection measures. Deceptively, these other oils will not be listed on the label, nor will most people be able to discern that their olive oil is not pure.

In 2016, *60 Minutes* did an exposé on the Italian olive oil industry and exposed that it has been corrupted by the Mafia. They are adding large amounts of cheap omega-6 vegetable oils, typically sunflower oils, and generating over $16 billion in sales a year as a result of the substitution. If at all possible, taste the oil before you buy it. While this won't necessarily be a guarantee of quality (especially if you're not skilled at picking out all the potentially subtle taste differences), it can help you to pick out the freshest-tasting oil possible. And if you open a bottle at home and find that it tastes rancid or "bad," return it to the store for a refund.

When you need an oil to cook with, coconut oil, *not* olive oil, is the ideal choice, because it is the only one that is stable enough to resist heat-induced damage. Extra virgin olive oil is excellent when used for cold dishes, but cooking with it is virtually guaranteed to damage this sensitive oil, as high temperatures can further degrade its molecular structure and create free radicals. However, it is important to understand that high-heat cooking with *any* oil, even coconut oil, will damage it. I personally use an induction burner to fry foods that allows me to cook foods as low as 100 degrees Fahrenheit, although I typically cook at 140 to 150.

Apart from its large amount of unsaturated fats that make it very prone to oxidative damage, extra virgin olive oil has a significant drawback even when used cold: it's still extremely perishable. It contains chlorophyll, which accelerates decomposition and makes the oil go rancid quite quickly.

Protein

In nature, nearly all animal protein sources are also sources of a significant amount of fat. In order to help you meet your daily fat allotment without exceeding your daily protein totals, avoid any low-fat dairy products or "lean" meats. Instead, seek to make the majority of your sources of protein high-fat options—chicken thighs with the skin on versus skinless chicken breast, for example.

As I outline in Chapter 9, you want to keep your protein intake at any given meal to 12 to 15 grams for women and 15 to 20 grams for men (assuming three meals per day). However, if you are immune compromised or recovering from surgery/illness or have higher physical activity demands, you will need about 25 percent more.

When I first learned of therapeutic high-fat diets, I simply didn't understand that anyone could fulfill their daily protein needs without overreliance on animal products—most of which have come from animals that have been raised on feedlots, which are degrading to the environment, the animals' quality of life, and the nutrient content of the meat they produce. (To be clear, I advocate eating certain animal products, but only those from pasture-raised animals that have no added hormones or antibiotics—look for the "American Grassfed" certification from the American Grassfed Association [AGA], which was just announced at the time of this writing.) Now I know better. Nuts and seeds are excellent sources of protein, with an average of 4 to 8 grams per ¼ cup, and most vegetables contain 1 to 2 grams of protein per ounce. With a target of 45 to 55 grams of protein in a day, plant sources can easily meet your protein needs.

Seafood

Seafood is the ideal source of the omega-3 fats EPA and DHA, but especially DHA, which is the single most important fat for your biological health. It is the only major fat that is not burned for fuel but integrated directly into your cellular and mitochondrial membranes.

As levels of pollutants in the water (including mercury) have increased, you have to be very choosy about which types of seafood you decide to eat. Among the least contaminated fish, and the highest in healthy omega-3 fat, are Alaskan and sockeye salmon. Neither is allowed to be farmed and they are therefore always wild caught. The risk of sockeye accumulating high amounts of mercury and other toxins is minimal given its short life span. Additionally, bioaccumulation of toxins is reduced because neither of these species of salmon feeds on smaller, highly contaminated fish.

The closer a fish is to the bottom of the food chain, the less contamination it will likely have accumulated in its lifetime, so other safe choices include small fish like sardines, anchovies, mackerel, and herring. Sardines are one of the most concentrated sources of omega-3 fats, with one serving containing more than 50 percent of your recommended daily value, making them one of the best dietary sources of animal-based omega-3s.[15] Just be sure to get your sardines in water, not olive oil, as nearly all the olive oil used to pack this fish is not fit for human consumption.

Avoid Farmed Fish

Although farmed salmon is more plentiful and cheaper than wild Alaskan salmon, I strongly discourage consumption of farmed salmon due to its inferior nutritional profile, environmental drawbacks, added dyes, and other potential health hazards.

Most important, it is almost 5 times higher in omega-6 fat, and the typical American already gets 10 to 20 times more omega-6 oils than they need. Overall, farmed salmon can contain anywhere from 14.5 to 34 percent fat, whereas wild salmon contains only 5 to 7 percent fat. Because many toxins accumulate most readily in fat, farmed salmon contains far more toxins than wild.

Farmed fish are also subject to many of the same issues as concentrated animal feeding operation (CAFO) beef and pork: namely, high antibiotic and pesticide use and GMO feed. Unfortunately, recent investigations by Oceana—an international organization focused on protecting our oceans created by a group of foundations including the Pew Charitable Trusts—have shown that as much as 80 percent of the fish marked as "wild" may actually be farmed, and that includes salmon. In restaurants, 90 to 95 percent of salmon is farmed, yet is often listed on the menu as "wild."[16]

Given these inaccurate representations, how can you tell whether your salmon fillet is wild or farmed? For one thing, the flesh of the salmon will give you a clue. Wild sockeye salmon is bright red, courtesy of its natural accumulation of astaxanthin, a powerful antioxidant. Sockeye salmon actually has one of the highest concentrations of natural astaxanthin found in any food.

Wild salmon is also very lean, so the fat marks—those white stripes you see in the meat—are quite thin. If a fish is pale pink (or dyed red) with wide fat marks, the salmon is likely farmed. Avoid Atlantic salmon, as these fish are almost always farmed.

Get Savvy about "Fake" Seafood

The seafood industry is rife with fraud. As Larry Olmsted points out in his excellent—if alarming—book *Real Food/Fake Food*, the vast majority of seafood sold in America isn't what it claims to be. As I mentioned, fish that is labeled wild is actually farmed. Or Chinese shrimp—which has consistently tested as being contaminated with harmful chemicals and is typically raised by what are essentially slave laborers—is passed off as coming from a different country. And restaurants often pass one fish off as another. For instance, red snapper is almost never actual red snapper: it'll be an inexpensive farmed fish like tilapia, probably imported from Southeast Asia, and probably farmed under dubious conditions.

"You could go out for a week and order red snapper every day and there's a good chance you're never going to get it," Olmsted told me when I interviewed him for my website.

A report by the ocean conservation group Oceana revealed that over 30 percent of shrimp products sold in U.S. grocery stores and restaurants are misrepresented.[17, 18] Fifteen percent were mislabeled in regard to production method (farm raised or wild caught) or species.

The ramifications of this frequent misrepresentation and mislabeling can be more serious than simply overpaying for an inferior product. In an earlier test published in 2013, Oceana discovered that 84 percent of white tuna sampled from U.S. retail outlets was actually escolar—a fish that can cause severe digestive problems (earning it the nickname "Ex-Lax fish").[19]

So how can you make sure you're actually getting what you're paying for? Here are a few strategies for buying seafood that is actually what it is purported to be:

- Buy your fish from a trusted local fishmonger or, surprisingly, a big-box retailer. This class of megastore has a lot of leverage in the industry and studies have shown that their labeling is highly accurate.

- When buying fish from grocery stores, look for third-party labels that verify quality, such as the Marine

Stewardship Council (its logo features the letters MSC and a blue checkmark in the shape of a fish). MSC has auditors who certify where the fish came from and how it got to you. Other labels that signify improved sustainability are Whole Foods Market Responsibly Farmed, Global Aquaculture Alliance Best Practices, Fishwise, and Seafood Safe.

- Look for Alaskan fish. Since Alaska doesn't permit aquaculture, all Alaskan fish is wild caught. The Alaskan fishing industry has some of the cleanest water and the best-maintained and most sustainable fisheries. To verify authenticity, look for the state of Alaska's "Wild Alaska Pure" logo. This is one of the more reliable ones, and it's a particularly good sign to look for if you're buying canned Alaskan salmon, which is less expensive than salmon steaks.

- *The Atlantic*[20] suggests buying your seafood from a member of the Better Seafood Bureau.[21] This trade organization reports fraud found along the seafood supply chain.

- You're also less likely to get scammed if you seek out seafood that has not been imported, as domestic fisheries tend to follow the rules for seafood labeling. Many coastal areas have seafood markets dedicated to fresh, high-quality seafood that is brought in daily. Here you can talk to the owner directly, who should be able to give you details about where the seafood came from.

- If you are going to eat shrimp, look for wild-caught shrimp from the Gulf of Mexico and a third-party certification that indicates the shrimp is from where it says it's from. Keep in mind that a minimum price per pound for shrimp is typically in excess of $18. If you see a deal that seems too good to be true, it almost certainly is.

- Last but not least, when possible, purchase the whole fish, as it's far more difficult to misrepresent the fish species when it's not cut up and filleted.

If you are a seafood lover and eating more types of fish and shellfish is important to you, use this list, compiled by the Natural Resources Defense Council, to select the least contaminated types.[22]

Least Mercury (Recommended)

- Anchovy
- Butterfish
- Catfish
- Clam
- Crab (domestic)
- Crawfish
- Croaker (Atlantic)
- Flounder
- Haddock (Atlantic)
- Hake
- Herring
- Jacksmelt (Silverside)
- Mackerel (North Atlantic, chub)
- Mullet
- Oyster
- Plaice
- Pollock
- Salmon (canned)
- Salmon (wild)
- Sardine

- Scallop
- Shrimp
- Sole (Pacific)
- Squid (calamari)
- Tilapia (not farmed; hard to find)
- Trout (freshwater)
- Whitefish
- Whiting

Moderate (Consume Moderately)

- Bass (saltwater, striped, black)
- Buffalo fish
- Carp
- Cod (Alaskan)
- Lobster
- Mahi mahi
- Monkfish
- Perch (freshwater)
- Sheepshead
- Skate
- Snapper
- Tilefish (Atlantic)
- Tuna (canned chunk light, skipjack)

High Mercury (Avoid)

- Croaker (white Pacific)
- Halibut (Atlantic, Pacific)
- Mackerel (Spanish, Gulf)
- Perch (ocean)

- Sablefish
- Sea bass (Chilean)
- Tuna (albacore, yellowfin)

Highest Mercury (Never Eat)

- Bluefish
- Grouper
- Mackerel (king)
- Marlin
- Orange roughy
- Shark
- Swordfish
- Tuna (bigeye, ahi)

Finally, no matter what type of fish you're considering, look for varieties that have received the Marine Stewardship Council certification, which assures that every component of the manufacturing process—from how the raw materials are harvested to how the product is manufactured—has been scrutinized by MSC and independently audited to ensure it meets sustainable standards.

DAIRY

Dairy can be classified as either high fat or high protein or a combination of both—while on MMT, you want to stick to the high-fat options. Some dairy products, such as milk and cottage cheese, are high in lactose (milk sugar), which is made up of a molecule of glucose bonded to a molecule of galactose. Once it's digested, the glucose will raise blood glucose levels. So limit your dairy consumption to the forms that are on the "high-fat dairy" list just below. And just as with your meat and eggs, you want to choose dairy that comes from grass-fed and organically raised cows—as with beef, look for the brand-new "American Grassfed" certification from the AGA. When available, raw dairy is preferable to pasteurized dairy. Even high-fat dairy contains some protein, so be sure to count those grams in your daily protein totals.

High-Fat Dairy (Okay in Moderation)

- Butter (12 grams of fat per tablespoon; minimal protein)
- Ghee (13 grams of fat per tablespoon; no protein)
- Heavy whipping cream (5 to 6 grams of fat per tablespoon; minimal protein)
- Cream cheese (4 to 5 grams of fat per tablespoon; some protein)
- Sour cream (2 to 3 grams of fat per tablespoon; some protein)
- Parmesan cheese (1.4 grams of fat per tablespoon; high protein—use all cheeses mainly as a condiment)
- Cheddar cheese (9 grams of fat per ounce; high protein)
- Brie cheese (8 grams of fat per ounce; high protein)

High-Protein Dairy (Avoid)

- Milk
- Cottage cheese
- Ricotta
- Yogurt
- Kefir

Note: High-fat dairy contains estrogen metabolites that may play a role in hormone-sensitive cancers, such as breast, uterine, ovarian, and prostate. Use dairy sparingly, if at all, if you have this type of cancer. Unless it is organic, it is likely contaminated with Roundup, hormones, antibiotics, and even worse, antibiotic-resistant bacteria.

Eggs

Despite the bad rap they've gotten from public health organizations and most mainstream media in the last decades, eggs are one of the healthiest foods you can eat, offering fantastic nutritional bang for your buck.

Many people, unfortunately, have been scared away from this healthy food source because eggs contain cholesterol, but it's becoming common knowledge that dietary cholesterol from natural sources poses no threat to your health (and may actually be beneficial). In 2015 the U.S. Dietary Guidelines removed the dietary cholesterol limit and added egg yolks to the list of suggested sources of protein. The long-overdue change came at the advice of the Dietary Guidelines Advisory Committee, which finally acknowledged what the science shows: that "cholesterol is not considered a nutrient of concern for overconsumption."[23]

Eggs provide the eight essential amino acids that your body requires to synthesize protein and that must be obtained through your diet because your body can't manufacture these amino acids on its own. Choose only true free-range organic eggs, also referred to as pasture raised, which come from hens that roam freely outdoors on an organic pasture where they can forage for their natural diet of seeds, worms, insects, and green plants.

It's important to remember that eggs have seven grams of protein, so you need to carefully integrate them into your diet to avoid consuming an excessive amount of protein that will in turn stimulate mTOR.

Tests have confirmed that pasture-raised eggs contain superior nutrients. Compared to eggs from CAFO chickens, they have:

- Two-thirds more vitamin A
- Three times more vitamin E
- Twice the omega-3 fatty acids
- Seven times more beta carotene

For a wide variety of reasons many people are very sensitive to chicken eggs but do very well on duck, quail, or goose eggs. If you're going to consume eggs regularly, it would be wise to broaden your variety and not just rely on chicken eggs. Also, be aware that raw eggs contain high levels of avidin, a protein that binds to the B vitamin biotin, and can lower biotin availability. So if you eat a lot of raw eggs, you may need to take a biotin supplement.

How you prepare your eggs also matters. Ideally, eat them raw or as close to raw as possible in order to keep the nutrients intact. Your risk of getting salmonella from eggs is always exceedingly slim. It may be slimmer still with pasture raised.

If you cannot eat them raw, poaching or soft-boiling (drizzling with MCT oil) is the next best option. Scrambled or fried eggs are the worst because the high heat oxidizes the cholesterol in the eggs, and could pose a problem if you are struggling with high cholesterol levels. Heating eggs also alters the chemical composition of the egg protein, which can then lead to allergic reactions or sensitivities. Eggs do contain a small amount of carbs, which should be counted in your daily carb totals.

NUTS AND SEEDS

Nuts and seeds are to the plant world what eggs are to the animal world, and are some of the most nutrient-dense foods on the planet. It's important to choose nuts that are organic, raw, and not irradiated, roasted in toxic oil, pasteurized, or coated in sugar or flavorings. Organic varieties are also free of antimicrobials and pesticides. Make sure they smell fresh and not musty, spoiled, stale, or rancid. These problems can also indicate the presence of fungal mycotoxins that are known to be damaging to your liver.

You should limit your overall intake of nuts to a few ounces a day and seeds to a few tablespoons per day to avoid overdosing on omega-6 fats. The best choices of nuts in your MMT plan are raw, organic macadamia nuts and pecans because they have the lowest amounts of carbs and protein and the highest amounts of fat. If you want to include other nuts, please confirm that they will not create an imbalance in your omega-6-to-omega-3 ratio.

Roasted nuts are tasty, but high heat is known to damage nutrients in nuts, including decreasing the availability of beneficial fats and amino acids.[24]

If you prefer to eat nuts and seeds roasted, roast them yourself so you can control temperature and time. For instance, raw pumpkin seeds can be sprinkled with Himalayan or other natural salt and then roasted on a low-heat setting in your oven for about 15 to 20 minutes—no more than 170 degrees Fahrenheit. This should minimize any heat-related damage.

A note of caution: Although nuts and seeds are excellent sources of nutrients and deserve a place in your MMT protocol, it is vital that you don't overeat them because they are also rich natural sources of omega-6 fats.

Omega-6 fats are essential to humans, but the reality is that you need *very little* of them in your diet. A major problem with processed oils high in omega-6 fats is that the oils are degraded during the refining process, so even naturally occurring omega-6 fats such as those that are in most nuts and seeds are unhealthy when consumed in excess because of their potential to be pro-inflammatory.

For example, when you eat too much of the most common omega-6 fatty acid, linoleic acid, unstable fatty acids get integrated into and disrupt your cardiolipin—a major lipid component of mitochondrial membranes. When mitochondrial cell membranes are compromised, mitochondrial metabolism and energy production is seriously impaired.[25] And please don't confuse linoleic with *linolenic,* as the latter is actually exactly what cardiolipin needs.

Thankfully, you can reduce the amount of linoleic acid that is integrated into your cardiolipin by substituting foods high in linoleic acid with omega-3 fats and the monounsaturated omega-9 fat oleic acid found in olive oil and many nuts, especially macadamia nuts, which are quite low in omega-6 fatty acids.

Linoleic acid's pro-inflammatory effect is not limited to mitochondrial membranes. In a 2013 study, excess linoleic acid appeared to exert a pro-inflammatory effect on cartilage. In patients with osteoarthritis, the presence of linoleic acid in the cartilage stimulated an inflammatory response, while oleic acid (monounsaturated) and palmitic acid (saturated) appeared to protect against cartilage destruction. This suggests that there may be a link between consuming high levels of linoleic acid and cartilage damage that leads to osteoarthritis.[26] For this and other reasons, take care not to exceed the recommended daily serving size of the seeds and nuts listed in this section.

The nuts and seeds I recommend for MMT include:

- Almonds (albeit in very limited amounts, as they are high in protein)
- Black cumin seeds
- Black sesame seeds
- Brazil nuts
- Raw cacao powder, nibs, and butter
- Chia seeds
- Flax seeds
- Macadamia nuts
- Pecans
- Psyllium seed husks
- Pumpkin seeds
- Sunflower seeds

For more information about these choices, including their nutrition and how to eat them, refer to Appendix B.

All other nuts not on this list are simply too high in protein for me to recommend using them. This is why they are not listed and should not be eaten on a regular basis.

It's important to look for nuts that are organic and raw, not irradiated, pasteurized, or coated in sugar. To avoid nuts that have been treated with antimicrobials and pesticides, choose organic varieties.

Part II

ADVANCED HEALING WITH MITOCHONDRIAL METABOLIC THERAPY

CHAPTER 6

BEFORE YOU START MMT

If you have read this far, you are likely ready to dive in and start reaping the health benefits of Metabolic Mitochondrial Therapy. But because precision matters with this plan, there are a few steps you need to take before you embark on a change. Doing so will pave the way to a smoother transition and ensure a higher rate of success in reaching your health goals. Work your way through the following actions. Some will be as easy as ordering a couple of crucial supplies; others, such as logging the food you eat, may take more resolve. By taking the time to take care of these things now, though, before you implement major dietary changes, you'll set yourself up for greater success when you are ready to embark on MMT in earnest.

Purchase a Few Choice Supplies

A Glucose Monitoring Device and Test Strips

One of the most important biometrics to track while implementing MMT is your blood glucose level. We have a diabetes epidemic in the U.S., with one in four having full-blown diabetes or pre-diabetes. As a result of the enormous monitoring demand, blood glucose monitors are relatively inexpensive and available without a prescription.

Most glucose meters range from $7 to $50 and are often discounted or free with coupons. The primary cost with testing your blood glucose comes from buying the strips. Test strips retail for anywhere between 25 cents to $2 a strip, depending on the brand and any technical features, such as linking to a computer program. That can get expensive if you check your blood glucose multiple times a day.

There are a wide variety of meters to choose from, but if you don't already have one, I have two recommendations that seem to be the favorites at the time of this writing. Keep in mind that technology is continually advancing, so do your own research; there may be better options for you when you read this. Amazon is an excellent resource to make these product comparisons and most of the prices I use in this section are taken from them.

- **Bayer Contour (Best for Inexpensive Glucose Monitoring Only)**

    For most people, the Bayer Contour system is the best choice because it is so economical. The monitor is under $10 and the strips are only 25 cents each.

- **Abbott Precision Xtra or Freestyle Optium Neo (For Both Glucose and Ketone Monitoring)**

    These devices are the best choices for monitoring blood ketones. They also measure your blood glucose levels, but both of them can be costly to use over the long term. It's not the cost of the device itself: at the time of this writing, the Precision Xtra costs $27 on Amazon.com and the Freestyle Optium costs $49.99. It's the cost of the strips. You'll need to use two different types of strips—one to measure glucose and one to measure ketones—and both types are relatively expensive. You can find glucose strips for these models that cost about 50 cents apiece, but you need to carefully select which ones you buy; there is a wide range, with many selling for nearly twice that price. The ketone test strips are much more expensive and cost around $4 to $6 for each strip. If you are serious about ketone monitoring, you can go to eBay and find ketone strips for your monitor at about half the price. Be careful when purchasing strips to look for the expiration date and make sure you will be able to use them before they expire. For this reason, even if you choose this device to monitor your ketones, I recommend you also purchase the Bayer Contour because it costs so much less per use, keeping your costs down over the long term.

Ketone Monitoring Devices and Accessories

There are three ways to measure your body's ketone output:

- **Blood test.** Devices that monitor ketones measure how much beta-hydroxybutyrate (BHB) is circulating in your blood. The best meters for this are those I mentioned that also test blood glucose levels: Abbott's Precision Xtra and Freestyle Optium Neo. While the initial investment is low, over time the cost of using either of these devices adds up as the ketone-measuring strips for each device are expensive, around $4 to $6 *per strip.*

- **Breathalyzer.** An effective and inexpensive long-term alternative to blood tests is a device that measures the acetone in your breath. In most cases the amount of acetone present in the breath correlates well with the amount of BHB present in the blood. You simply blow into the meter for 20 to 30 seconds and it will flash one of three different colors a specific number of times to indicate your level of ketosis. Breath ketone analyzers involve an initial investment. For example, Ketonix.co sells its version for $150—but the advantage is that you don't need to pay for testing strips and you don't have to draw any blood, so it is the best long-term solution. I personally do one or two Ketonix checks most days, especially when I am changing my program and need to confirm my level of ketosis.

- **Urine test.** For many decades, urine test strips that measure the presence of acetoacetate have been the most common way to measure ketosis. Perhaps you remember them from the days of the Atkins Diet movement. The reactive pad at the end of the strips remains beige if there are no ketones present and turns pink with light ketones and purple for strong ketones. But since they only detect acetoacetate and not BHB, the fuel preferred by most cells, urine tests provide limited insight into whether your body is actually burning fat for fuel. On the other hand, they're inexpensive, fairly convenient to use, and don't require pricking your finger. You can use the strips simply to see if your body is producing ketones (any level of pink color means that it is), but don't put too much stock in the results.

When to Monitor Ketones

Here are some guidelines to help you know when it's worth the effort to check in on your ketone levels:

- **At the start.** It's important to remember that you really only need to monitor your ketones closely at the beginning of your MMT journey. Doing so can provide you with important feedback in two areas: first, it will help you determine when you have successfully made the transition to burning fat, and second, it will help you fine-tune your personal limit on how many and what kind of carbs you can eat and still remain in that fat-burning state. You'll know you've made the transition to fat burning when your blood ketone levels are between 0.5 and 3.0 mmol/L. It can take some fine-tuning of your diet to get your numbers into this range, and monitoring your ketone levels can give you some very important quantifiable data on how well your plan is working.

- To get an accurate picture of how many carbs you can eat and still produce ample ketones, you'll want to stick to a specific number of carb grams to eat for two or three days—say, 30 to 40 grams—and then measure your ketones on each of those days to get an average. Then choose a different carb threshold, such as 40 grams, for two or three days and test again. The feedback you get on how many carbs produce the level of ketones you want will help you customize MMT to your own body. This customization is an essential component of the program. Your carb threshold is dynamic, so periodically performing this testing will help you adapt your intake to meet your body's changing needs.

- Generally, the longer you are in ketosis, the more metabolically flexible you become, which is the ultimate goal. So, if you are kicked out of ketosis in the initial few weeks, it might take you another week or longer to get back on track. Once you have fully made the transition to burning fat for fuel, what I call being "fat adapted," this switch happens much more easily.

  The ultimate goal is achieving the metabolic flexibility you had as a healthy child! Kids go very easily into ketosis even when they eat large amounts of net carbs. By the time you reach adulthood, you have likely been following a high-net-carb diet for decades and your body has lost its ability to easily switch in to fat-burning mode. By adopting MMT, you can gain that metabolic flexibility back.

- **When you make substantial changes in your food choices.** Once you achieve fat burning and have maintained it for a few weeks to a month, you really only need to check your ketone levels if you make changes to your diet—for example, in response to a stressful event, a change in routine, or a long period of travel. At those times, you want to be sure that you are still burning plenty of fat for fuel. Test once a day until you are certain that your ketone levels have returned to their previous range.

- **If you notice a rise in your blood glucose levels.** Should you notice your blood glucose numbers trending upward, it's time to get back to regular ketone testing for at least a few days. I recommend testing three times a day, including first thing in the morning, after lunch, and before bed. If your ketones are still in a good range, the change in glucose levels may be due to beneficial changes in insulin signaling. If your ketones are also low, it's likely that you are either eating too many carbs or too much protein. Experiment with reducing your carbs for two or three days and keep testing. Then do the same experiment with your protein consumption. See which strategy is more effective in getting your ketones up and your blood glucose down, and adjust your food intake accordingly.

- **As a way to monitor your long-term progress.** Ideally, you would check your ketone levels once or twice a week over the long term, choosing different times of the day. This is more important if you have a serious health condition that you are seeking to manage, but keeping a very loose check-in schedule will give you the feedback and motivation you need to keep going. Anything more than once or twice a week when you're *not* experiencing one of the situations I've just listed above is overkill.

Lancets and a Lancet-Holding Device

Whichever monitor you choose, you'll also need lancets and a lancet-holding device in order to draw a drop of blood. Lancets are around $5 for a box of 100, and the devices are well under $10. There is no major difference that I am aware of between brands, so merely obtain and use whatever ones are convenient for you. The one that comes with the Bayer Contour system will work just fine.

There is one major trick for using the lancet device: it is important to obtain a fairly significant drop of blood *before* you insert the test strip into your monitor. If the blood drop is too small, or you approach it from an oblique angle, it won't absorb rapidly enough and you will get a false reading. This is always something to consider if you get an unexpectedly high reading. In these cases it is best to obtain another drop of blood and use a new test strip to take another reading. Experiment with testing blood glucose first before you test ketones. You'll need a much bigger drop of blood for ketones and you don't want to waste even one strip!

A Digital Food Scale

As I'll cover a little later in this chapter, an integral part of MMT is using a tool that allows you to track your food intake. When you do this, it is nearly always advisable to use weight measurements (in grams), especially for small amounts. The most common mistake people make is to guess at the amounts of the foods they eat and enter those guesses into the food diary. For example, rather than estimating a tablespoon of seeds as one-half ounce, you need to weigh them on a scale. I made this mistake when I first embarked on MMT. Once I realized my tallies were off and started weighing instead of just measuring my seeds, I found a tablespoon of psyllium was only 4 grams, while a tablespoon of cacao nibs weighed nearly three times that, at 11 grams.

So if you don't already have an electronic digital kitchen food scale, plan on purchasing one soon. Prices start at under $20. Make sure to purchase one that measures up to a few pounds or kilos. These are typically accurate to 1 gram. If you need more precision, you can purchase scales that are accurate to 0.1 grams for about the same cost. Just be sure that they will still weigh a large quantity.

All digital scales have a tare function, also known as auto-zero, which means it automatically deducts the weight of the container you're using if it's placed on the scale before you turn it on. That way, you are only measuring the weight of the food and not the plate or container. Then just place what you need to weigh into the container or onto the plate and enter that weight in grams into Cronometer.com (the online tool I recommend to track your food intake and give you invaluable feedback on how well you're feeding your body—much more on this later in this chapter).

Measuring Spoons

You will want to have a set or two of stainless steel measuring spoons so you can accurately measure out the food you then weigh on your digital scale.

Establish a Baseline with These Lab Tests

Although the dietary changes I outline in this book will dramatically improve your health, it is important to understand that there are two factors that will limit your improvement: insufficient vitamin D levels and too much iron. That is why I strongly encourage you to initially measure vitamin D and iron levels before you start and seek to optimize them at the same time you are starting the diet.

I believe these two tests are absolutely essential to optimize your health, as you simply are unable to perceive your vitamin D and iron levels without them, and these levels have enormous influence on your mitochondrial health. I also recommend a mercury analysis to screen for high levels of this prevalent and harmful toxin.

I also recommend three additional tests described below that monitor your health and are wise to take before you get started so you can see how much improvement you make after you successfully implement the program.

Vitamin D

Vitamin D is, without question, the most important nutrient that the majority of people are consistently deficient in. Low vitamin D levels are caused in large part by a lack of sun exposure, either because of living in locations that do not have enough direct sunshine throughout the year or simply not exposing large surfaces of your skin to the sun on a regular basis. Age and skin tone also affect how much vitamin D is synthesized in your skin.

You should have this test performed at least once a year, and perhaps every few months, until you develop a routine that will ensure you maintain optimal vitamin D levels—which fall in the 40 to 60 ng/mL range. There are two tests for vitamin D; you need to ask for the 25-hydroxyvitamin D, also referred to as 25-(OH)D. There is not enough room in this book to review all the benefits and means of achieving an optimized vitamin D level. You can review my website, mercola.com, or my last book, *Effortless Healing*, for those details.

For now, know that the ideal way to optimize your vitamin D level is through sensible sun exposure. You may need to modify your routine to make this possible. Vitamin D supplements are a poor substitute for sun exposure but can be a practical reality for many whose circumstances prevent them from optimal sun exposure for long stretches of time during the year. Most people don't understand that vitamin D is actually a biomarker for ultraviolet B exposure, which has other actions other than making vitamin D. So when you provide your body with oral vitamin D but no sun exposure, you miss out on many important, but likely as yet unrecognized, benefits of optimal solar exposure.

I personally take this issue very seriously and moved to a subtropical area so I can get vitamin D from the sun year round the way we were designed to, from safe solar exposure. I have not taken any vitamin D supplements for nearly 10 years yet have maintained optimal vitamin D levels. Living in a state where the sun shines frequently, I make it a priority to spend time outside in the sun. So I schedule my work around my solar exposures, and most every day I am able to spend one to three hours walking in the sun on the beach. In the winter, when there isn't much UV available, I walk at noon. In the summer I walk early in the morning, as the UV exposures and temperatures are too high during midday. To justify this much time outside, I read on my Kindle and am able to read about 150 books a year.

Ferritin

Checking your iron levels is easy and can be done with a simple blood test called a serum ferritin test. The test measures the carrier molecule of iron, a protein found inside cells called ferritin, which stores the iron. If your ferritin levels are low, it means your iron levels are also low.

As I outlined in Chapter 4, I believe this is one of the most important tests you can have done regularly as part of a preventive, proactive health screening. This is especially true if you are an adult male or a postmenopausal woman who is no longer losing blood through your monthly menstrual cycle.

Please refer to Chapter 4 to learn more why this test is so important.

Mercury Analysis

Most of us are contaminated with mercury as it is prevalent in most seafood, and in silver mercury amalgam fillings. There are many tests for mercury levels out there but, in my experience, the best test is one that detects where the mercury is coming from, and the only test that I know that does that is from Quicksilver Scientific (https://www.quicksilverscientific.com/mercury-testing/testing/mercury-tri-test).

Optional but Highly Recommended Blood Tests

You don't need these tests before you start on the MMT plan, but you should have these labs drawn when you can; they will give you an important baseline. You can have them done again after you've adopted MMT for a few months and check to see that your numbers are moving in the right direction.

- **Fasting Insulin.** Measuring your insulin will provide powerful insights into how effectively you are burning fat. The test must be done fasting or you will not have accurate feedback. The lower the number is, the better. Ideally the level should be below 2 to 3 mIU/L. Levels over 5 suggest you are not burning fat as your primary fuel.

- **Fasting Lipid Panel.** Our culture is obsessed with cholesterol levels, to the point that one in four adults in the U.S. take a statin drug to lower cholesterol levels. Nevertheless, elevated cholesterol levels are rarely a risk factor for heart disease, although elevated triglycerides clearly are. Fortunately, elevated triglycerides can easily be corrected by this program and lowered to an ideal level of below 75. The triglyceride-to-HDL ratio is also helpful and should be below 2. You can also look at the HDL-to-cholesterol ratio, which should be above 24 percent—the higher the number, the better on this measure.

- **HS-CRP.** This test measures the amount of a protein called C-reactive protein (CRP) in your blood. CRP measures general levels of inflammation in your body. There are two types, the regular test and the high sensitivity test (HS). It is best to get the more sensitive HS test done to measure CRP levels, which ideally should be below 0.7 mg/L.

Record Your Starting Body Measurements

To get to where you want to go, it's important to have a clear picture of the point where you started. Taking the time now to analyze and record a few specific measurements—known as "biometrics"—will do two important things:

- It will help inspire you to make changes. When you can quantify key markers of your health, and objectively see where you stand now, it will motivate you to commit to doing things differently.

- It will give you a way to see your progress. It is incredibly rewarding to see your numbers start to improve and to know that the choices you're making are producing measurable results.

These are the measurements I recommend you take as baselines. You can also input and track these at Cronometer.com, a fantastic online resource for tracking food intake and much more that I explain in detail at the end of this chapter.

Body Fat Percentage

Body fat is essential to your health. It protects your organs and stores energy and vital nutrients (think of the fat-soluble vitamins A, D, E, and K). Have too little of it, and your body can turn to muscle protein for fuel and enter what's known as a catabolic state. On the other hand, too much body fat—especially visceral fat—is part of a deadly epidemic. It is linked to chronic diseases including heart disease, diabetes, and cancer. It's important to keep your body fat percentage within healthy ranges—so important, in fact, that it's not something you want to leave to chance. I strongly recommended that you use the most accurate body fat assessing method that is available to you. (I will describe several below.)

How much fat you are carrying in your body is a vital gauge of your current metabolic health. Knowing your body fat percentage also allows you to calculate your lean body mass, which is essentially all parts of your body that aren't fat. Knowing your lean body mass will help you calculate precisely how much protein you should be eating on a daily basis, another crucial metric that will help you enormously in your quest for optimal health (and one I will discuss in more detail in Chapter 7).

Once you determine your body fat percentage, subtract it from 100 to determine your percentage of lean body tissue. From there, multiply that percentage by your current weight to get your total amount of lean body mass. For example, let's say that you use one or more of the methods I list below to learn that you have 30 percent body fat. That means you have 70 percent lean body tissue. Then you take 70 percent of your total body weight (multiply it by 0.7) to get your lean body mass.

There are several ways to determine how much body fat you are carrying. Each has its pluses and minuses. I've listed them below in order of cost, complexity, and accuracy, from lowest to highest:

- **Photo approximation.** The easiest and least expensive way to gauge your body fat percentage is to take a photo of yourself in your underwear (the most painful part) and then compare it to photos of people at different body fat percentages. You can find the photos for comparison on Cronometer.com or by doing an Internet search for "body fat percentage" and selecting the Images tab on the results page. Of course, this isn't the most accurate method, as it requires you to be objective about your appearance, but it can give you a general idea of where you are and what the next stage in personal health actually looks like.

- **Skin calipers.** This low-tech method involves using an inexpensive, lightweight handheld device known as a skin caliper to measure the thickness of a fold of your skin and the fat that lies beneath it. Calipers cost anywhere from a couple of dollars to a couple of hundred dollars and resemble a small pair of tongs. They can measure distance down to a millimeter. They can readily be purchased on Amazon and come with comprehensive instructions and formulas that will calculate your body fat percentage. Or you can ask your doctor if he or she can measure this for you.

  Taken at specific locations on your body, caliper readings can help you determine the total percent of body fat. Although there is always the possibility of error, body fat calipers are one of the most time-tested and accurate ways to measure body fat. For results to be truly helpful, it's best to engage the help of another person—particularly for women, who need to measure the skin fold on the back of the upper arm, a difficult-to-reach area—and to use that same person to take your measurements each time. You'll also need to either perform some simple calculations on your own or use an online calculator developed for just this purpose to translate those measurements into your body fat percentage.

- **Bioelectrical impedance analysis (BIA).** This approach can be as simple as stepping on a specific type of scale that measures body fat, readily available online for about $50. BIA sends an electrical signal through your body, where it will pass easily through lean body mass—which is up to 75 percent water, a good conductor of electricity—but be impeded by your fat tissue, which contains low amounts of water. While this analysis is certainly convenient, there is some concern that it may not be as accurate in nutritional ketosis because making the switch to fat-burning has a diuretic effect. This is because every molecule of glycogen is stored with 3 to 4 grams of water, so when you burn through your glycogen stores on your way to fat-burning, you also release water weight and this may throw off the accuracy of BIA.[1] This measurement, along with other factors—such as your height, weight, age, and sex, which you enter into the device—is then used to calculate your percentage of body fat, lean body mass, and other body composition measurements. Although the absolute value may be off a bit, a BIA scale is very accurate and typically very consistent. Even though the number itself might not be correct, it will accurately measure your body fat day-to-day variability, which is a far more reliable monitor than your body weight.

- **Skulpt (electrical impedance myography, or EIM).** EIM, which was developed by a professor of neurology at Harvard Medical School, is a relatively new technology. Devices using EIM only recently came to market, although they have been tested in hospitals for over a decade. This method is similar to BIA in that it uses electricity to determine certain qualities of your body tissue.

  An EIM device, such as the Skulpt Aim Fitness Tracker—a handheld gadget about the size of a pack of cigarettes that you hold on a few different sites on your body—uses a current that is optimized to flow through fat as well as provide feedback about the quality of your muscles. It is also designed to be placed on specific muscles throughout the body, giving a detailed picture of how strong each muscle group is and gathering specific fat readings from multiple parts of your body.

  The Skulpt Aim claims to be three times more accurate than skin fold calipers and five times more

accurate than bioimpedance. It is relatively expensive—
the device costs $149—although it can be shared with
family members, friends, or clients. Skulpt is also coming
out with a more basic model, the Chisel, that also reads
body fat percentage and muscle quality and that at the
time of this writing is retailing for $99.

- **Bod Pod (air displacement plethysmography).** This
  option involves sitting inside an egg-shaped compart-
  ment for five minutes or less as instruments measure
  how much air your body displaces. Although you will
  need to sit still, there's no discomfort associated with the
  test; some people report the feeling as similar to being in
  an elevator or in a plane that has just taken off. The Bod
  Pod is one of the most accurate body composition tests
  available today. The only issue is that you will need to
  find a Bod Pod near you (visit http://www.bodpod.com/
  en/cosmed-offices to search for locations), and a single
  visit generally costs around $50. Also, you will need
  follow-up visits to determine if there have been changes
  in your body composition since your initial visit.

- **DEXA scan (dual-energy X-ray absorptiometry).** A
  DEXA scan is an X-ray that gives a detailed reading of
  overall and regional fat mass, lean mass, and bone mass;
  you may be familiar with it, particularly if you are a
  woman, as this method is frequently used to measure
  bone density. Although it is considered by many to be
  very accurate in measuring body fat, Dr. Jason Fung
  finds that it falsely measures lean body mass.

  The use of X-rays makes this method the most
  accurate on this list. It also makes the DEXA scan one
  of the most expensive methods, as well as a source of
  exposure to radiation, although at very minor levels.
  You'll likely have to do a little digging to find a place
  to have the scan done—many hospitals, universities
  with exercise physiology centers, and health care facil-
  ities have one—and then you'll have to pay anywhere

from $50 to $150 or more for the scan. Keep in mind that for a DEXA scan to be truly helpful, you'll need to repeat it in a few months to see how your body composition has changed. (Make it very clear when you make your appointment that you want to test for lean body mass, not bone density.)

Waist Size

Measuring your waist size is an important metric to track, as waist size is a fairly accurate benchmark for predicting your risk of death from a heart attack and other causes. It is also a quick and easy measurement to take: with a tape measure, measure the distance around the smallest area of your abdomen, below your rib cage and above your belly button. There are inexpensive tape measures available that lock into place around your waist and then self-retract, taking any guesswork out of how tightly or loosely to hold the tape and making it even easier to read your measurement. Search for "MyoTape" on the Internet to find one.

The following is a general guide for healthy waist circumference:

- Men: 37 to 40 inches is overweight; greater than 40 inches is obese

- Women: 31.5 to 34.6 inches is overweight; greater than 34.6 inches is obese

Your waist size is such an important predictor of health because the type of fat that is stored around your waistline—called "visceral fat" or "belly fat"—is related to the release of proteins and hormones that cause inflammation, which can in turn damage your arteries and affect how you metabolize sugars and fats. For this reason, visceral fat is strongly linked to type 2 diabetes, heart disease, stroke, Alzheimer's, and other chronic diseases. Seeing your waist size come down is a great indicator of improving health.

General Body Fat Percentage Guidelines from the American Council on Exercise

Classification	Women (% fat)	Men (% fat)
Essential Fat	10–13%	2–5%
Athletes	14–20%	6–13%
Fitness	21–24%	14–17%
Acceptable	25–31%	18–24%
Obese	32% and higher	25% and higher

Weight

I am listing total weight last because, on its own, it is not a very accurate marker of health. Your weight has many variables, including the density of your bone structure. So, for example, a lean, muscular football player may weigh a lot, but that certainly doesn't mean they have a high risk of metabolic dysfunction. Still, your weight is easy to measure and track and can give you good information on which direction you are trending.

I recommend you take a starting weight and then weigh yourself daily at the same time of the day, typically after you have had your morning bowel movement and before you eat your first meal. This will help to minimize daily variations. Know, though, that it is possible to weigh more than you used to if you are gaining weight as muscle at the same time that you are losing fat. So take your weight measurement with a grain of salt and resist the temptation to weigh yourself several times throughout the day.

Sign Up with and Start Using Cronometer.com

Without an accurate analytical tool for tracking food intake, it will be virtually impossible to assess and fine-tune your program. Flying blind simply will not provide you with a comprehensive understanding of what you are actually eating, either in terms of calories or nutrients.

More importantly, you won't be able to determine the balance of macronutrients that's best for you; you won't know, for instance, how many grams of protein keep you in the fat-burning zone if you don't know how many grams of protein you need or eat. From my perspective it is absolutely imperative that you consistently use a tool like the online nutrient trackers I mention below if you are going to have any hope of successfully implementing this program.

Entering the foods you eat into an online database will allow you to keep an accurate record of everything you eat or drink. You can then combine this nutrient information with the biometric data that you collect—such as your weight and blood glucose levels—so you can understand how the foods you choose to eat are affecting your biochemistry and metabolism.

Fortunately there is a great tool that I initially learned about through one of the readers of my health newsletter. Cronometer.com is a free online service with three major advantages:

- **Data accuracy.** Cronometer is committed to using only high-quality macro- and micronutrient data that are obtained from the most reliable sources so you get an accurate record of your nutritional intake. Cronometer obtains most of its data from the USDA National Nutrient Database and the Nutrition Coordinating Center Food and Nutrient Database.

  Cronometer has added commercial food products to its databases, but these entries are limited to the nutrition details listed on the label, which will not include many of the micronutrients that are important to your health. For example, Brazil nuts are an excellent source of selenium. But if you enter "Trader Joe's Brazil Nuts," you will not see how much selenium you're taking in as it's not listed on the nutrition label. You're better off entering the generic "Brazil nuts" from the USDA, which provides data on all of the known nutrients for Brazil nuts. The same goes for the bar code scanner in the mobile app; these items only contain the label nutrition facts. So while it's very convenient to be able to log items with a bar code scanner, I only recommend doing so if you can't find an equivalent food from the higher-quality data sources.

All items in the database contain macronutrient information so you can see at a glance how many grams of carb, protein, and fat you're taking in. So if you aren't concerned with micronutrient tracking, you can be more relaxed about logging items from the less complete data sources and bar code scanner.

- **Elegant, easy-to-use graphical interface.** To make data entry easier, you can create your own custom recipes so you can easily add multiple ingredients with one click. For example, my three regular meals each have over 15 ingredients but I can enter the entire recipe as a "food" on the diary page with just one click. Setting up these customized recipes may take some time initially, but once it is done, data entry will typically take you less than two minutes a day.

  The real power of this program comes from the detailed graphs that show you exactly how close you come to meeting your personalized nutrient goals, down to the individual amino acids, vitamins, and minerals. You can tell Cronometer to set a dynamic macronutrient target for you that lines up with MMT by choosing the "High Fat/Ketogenic" option in the pop-up box that opens when you click on "Calories Summary." When you do that, you will see a colored bar in the center of your dashboard that displays at a glance both the grams and the percentage of each macronutrient you consumed that day.

  Many of the metrics in your dashboard also unveil further detail in pop-up displays if you hover your mouse over them. For example, you can mouse over the "Fat" bar and it will show you the precise percentage of monounsaturated, polyunsaturated, and saturated fats. Or, you can mouse over any other nutrient meter (such as carbs or fiber) and it will show you the top ten foods in that category so you aren't just guessing about your intake.

This is a convenient way to quickly identify the foods that are contributing to your nonfiber carbohydrates and protein totals for the day.

- **Allows you to keep a visual record of your progress** via a feature called "Snapshots," where you can upload body fat percentage photos of yourself at different times during your MMT journey and see the changes that occur in your physical appearance.

- **Only food tracker customized for MMT.** The founder of the Cronometer, Aaron Davidson, actually developed the program for his own use because none of the existing trackers provided him with enough of the information he thought was important to his health. Aaron is a passionate anti-aging advocate and wanted a tool that could easily help him implement his own nutrition program—so he created his own! I have included the story of his experience with the program below.

Now for the best part: I contacted Aaron and asked him to customize Cronometer for those seeking to implement MMT and he was very willing to do that. The result is a program that is unlike any other on the planet. It will help empower you to dramatically improve your health. It will also serve to advance nutrition research by allowing us to anonymously pool nutrition data from the records of people who are implementing MMT.

You can go to https://cronometer.com/mercola/ to sign up for your free Cronometer account and to enroll in the MMT study. MMT users will also be eligible for a 20 percent discount on all Cronometer gold subscriptions.

Discovering an Even More Effective—and Enjoyable—Way to Optimize Health

By Aaron Davidson, creator of cronometer.com

I originally wrote the program for Cronometer in 2005 because I was following the CRON (Calorie Restriction with Optimal Nutrition) diet. CRON requires eating very few calories while still attempting to get all your required nutrition from high-quality foods. It's nearly impossible to practice without software to carefully track and put together nutritious food combinations on a very tight caloric budget. Hundreds of studies have shown that a CRON diet can have powerful anti-aging effects. It is, however, very difficult to maintain. I managed to follow it for several years, but eventually gave it up.

Then I began to hear more and more about the research on ketogenic (high-fat, low-carb) diets and intermittent fasting, both of which share a great deal of benefits with caloric restriction. The difference is that intermittent fasting and fat-burning diets are much easier to practice than the CRON diet.

Many people adopt a high-fat, low-carb diet in order to lose weight or to treat a disease such as cancer, diabetes, or epilepsy. I had no chronic conditions. I was in good shape. But I am passionate about working toward optimal health. I was swayed by the mounting evidence that a ketogenic diet can reduce oxidative stress, normalize hormonal balances, lower inflammation, and increase mental clarity and focus.

I'm also a huge nerd, and to be honest, having an excuse to test and track my ketone and blood glucose levels every day was just the sugar-free icing on top. I find it fascinating to see my body's response to various foods and eating schedules. By carefully tracking my food intake and measuring blood ketones and glucose, I have learned what my maximum carbohydrate threshold is for me to stay in ketosis. One bummer: I learned that enjoying a beer meant no more ketones the next day!

At the same time I started eating a low-carb, high-fat diet, I also started practicing intermittent fasting. I do both multiday fasts (allowing only water, coffee, tea, and broth) and daily fasting by constraining my eating window to seven hours. At the start, fasting was very difficult, but as I've become fat adapted it has become far easier. I've learned the importance of a bit of broth through the day to keep electrolytes balanced, which makes a huge difference.

Some of my favorite side effects of the fat-burning lifestyle include:

- Steady mental energy all day. No mid-afternoon crash!

- I rarely feel hungry between meals.

- My chronic gingivitis has vanished.

One thing I do allow, since I'm not practicing this diet for any sort of critical medical condition, is to periodically take a break around the holidays. I don't recommend doing this unless you have a very disciplined personality. I will spend a few months in keto mode, take a few weeks enjoying the social eating that comes with holidays, indulge in some of the "off limits" foods, and then restart back into keto mode with a multiday fast. For me, it's a lifestyle choice—I want to spend the majority of my time in a fat-burning state and still have some flexibility to switch off a few times a year. It makes it easier for me to say no to the beer, pizza, and burgers during my strict keto periods if I know there will be time to enjoy these things at a later date. I don't feel deprived.

All told, I really enjoy the ketogenic lifestyle, and the food is great—bacon and eggs, fat bombs, nuts, salads drowned in olive oil, guacamole, creamy and coconut-y Thai stews. It's delicious!

How to Use Cronometer for MMT

To start, you can enter each food you eat separately, recording how much you ate in grams. It is important to actually measure here using an inexpensive digital kitchen scale and not just guess. Remember, the accuracy of your analysis will only be as valid as the data you enter.

Later on, when you have some favorite go-to meals, you can enter them as your own personal recipes. You can also enter favorite recipes that you create on your own or find online or in keto cookbooks.

That way, you can enter an entire meal with one click. You can add to this list at any time, but having your go-to meals already entered will make recording your daily intake quick and easy. Then, each morning, enter all the foods you plan to eat later that day, using it like a "planner."

This gives you the opportunity to view that day's analysis at the front end, *before* you eat it. It also gives you the flexibility to add or delete foods or change portion sizes to better reach your targets. This is far superior to entering the data after the fact, since you have lost the opportunity to make different choices that could have gotten you closer to your targets. So my advice to you is to always enter your data in the morning before you begin to prepare your meals.

Along these lines, it is important to point out the obvious: You need to enter *every* bit of food or drink that passes your lips. If you are inconsistent, or your entries don't reflect your actual portion sizes, then the data generated will be flawed and potentially damaging to your health.

It is *far* better to be honest and record everything, even if you regret your choice as soon as you make it. That way, you can learn from experience by noting exactly how your body responded to your choice, for example, by testing your postprandial rise in glucose. Failing to track accurately and completely makes it virtually impossible to make sense of your data. Remember, the only person you hurt by not accurately recording what you eat is yourself. Although I may sound overly dramatic, this could mean the difference between life and death, especially for those people who are using this program to manage diet as part of a cancer treatment strategy.

You can also tell Cronometer how much of a certain type of food you want to consume and it will help you keep track of how well you're adhering to these targets. It's called "setting your macronutrient targets," which I cover in more detail in Chapter 7. Cronometer's High Fat/Ketogenic option is a special case. Instead of targeting specific ratios, we dynamically calculate a maximum target for your carbohydrate and protein intake, and set the remainder to fats. This is because eating too many carbohydrates

Before You Start MMT

will suppress nutritional ketosis, and too much protein will do the same because the body can convert excess protein into glucose through gluconeogenesis.

Total Carbs versus Net Carbs

You can choose to track carbohydrates as total carbs or net carbs. By default we use net carbs: total carbs with fiber subtracted. This leads to more accurate calorie targets for carbs since fiber does not contribute heavily to your total calories.

Some nutrients, like vitamin D, are only found in small amounts in the foods you eat. After tracking your nutrient intake for a few days, you will see how deficient you are. Also keep in mind that the recommended daily allowance (RDA) for vitamin D is set at a ridiculously low level, so you'll want to be sure that you're getting at least three times the RDA for that nutrient. This usually means you'll need to supplement with D3. You will also be able to see which other specific nutrients are lacking in your diet. You can either shift your diet to foods that will help, or decide to take specific nutritional supplements (there is more on monitoring your vitamin D on page 117).

Although your identity will always remain private, the terms of service for using Cronometer allow us to anonymously compile the data to document MMT's effectiveness. The intention is to publish this data so we can prove to the world how effective this program really is.

Remember: If you choose to forego weighing your food, your results will not be accurate. So please, weigh all your foods before you enter the data. You typically will only need to weigh each food once because a tablespoon of the same food should always weigh the same. Weighing is not as much of an inconvenience as it may seem—in fact, you may even enjoy doing this, and it is an essential part of the process if you are going to obtain useful information from the program.

ADJUST YOUR MIND-SET

I want to address the mental and emotional aspects of embarking on MMT. It doesn't matter how much information you have if you are approaching any major life change without an open mind and an open heart because you will be limiting your opportunities for success. Why waste time on false starts?

The research shows that a fat-burning diet can trigger important and powerful changes in your health in just a few days. Having both the information *and* the inspiration you need will help you make the most of your entry into the fat-burning lifestyle. A positive attitude will help you attain, and build on, these benefits from the very start.

You may have picked up this book because you are facing a serious medical diagnosis, whether it's something acute, like late-stage cancer, or chronic, such as diabetes, weight-loss challenges, or fibromyalgia.

Wherever you may fall on the spectrum between healthy and ill, there is a fundamental shift in thinking that needs to precede action. And that is to start viewing yourself as an active and empowered participant in your own health care.

This is a departure from the way the conventional medical system currently operates. It views patients as being recipients of care—meaning the doctors make the decisions and you follow along. This dynamic isn't merely the result of physician arrogance. Instead, many patients are understandably frightened and overwhelmed, and are seeking a "magic bullet" that is simple, quick, and effective; submitting 100 percent to a physician's care involves minimal effort and maximal faith. Instead of taking an active role in their health care decisions, these patients merely want doctors to "fix" them, to map out the "best" course of action, and to know the next best step at any given juncture.

Looping Your Doctors in on Your MMT Journey

If you've read this far, you clearly are seeking to do something different. You are educating yourself about proven ways to take on more responsibility for and control of your own health. But now that we are getting past research and into actual implementation, you may need to step up your resolve to become an active decision maker on your health journey.

A big piece of adopting the fat-burning diet is seeing yourself as a copilot—because you absolutely want your conventional doctors to be informed about what you are doing. Although you don't need their permission to change your diet—any more than you would need their permission to eat pizza for dinner—you do want everyone who participates in your health care to be aware of the actions you are taking on your own behalf, including everything from food plans to supplements to complementary care (such as acupuncture, chiropractic, massage, or other holistic health modalities).

There are two major reasons they need to be informed. First, there may be elements of your particular situation that need to be closely monitored (see the sidebar on page 136 for a list). And second, if your doctors know about your change in diet, even if they don't believe it will have benefits, they can't deny the changes they see in you. This may not change their adherence to evidence-based protocols, but it may change their attitude about supporting your efforts. Hopefully, the changes they see in you will also encourage them to take this plan more seriously and research it for themselves—and perhaps even open their eyes to the power of food to treat illness.

Some Conditions That Require Medical or Nutritional Oversight during the Transition to MMT

- Liver cancer

- Elevated liver enzymes

- Esophageal surgery and/or radiation

- Head/neck radiation

- Diabetes

- Thyroid imbalances (hypothyroidism, hyperthyroidism, or Hashimoto's disease)

- Gastric bypass surgery or current lap band

- Impaired digestion, whether due to opioid use, neuromuscular disorders, neurodegenerative diseases, other illness, or side effects of medical treatment

- Food allergies, sensitivities, or aversions

- Leaky gut

- History of pancreatitis

- Family or personal history of kidney stones

- History of GI issues, such as IBS, Crohn's disease, or ulcerative colitis

- Renal disease

- Feeding tubes

- Gallbladder obstruction or removal. One can easily compensate for the lack of a gallbladder though with the use of lipase and ox bile supplements. So a gallbladder removal does not eliminate one from using a high fat diet.

- Low body weight

- Cancer cachexia

- Abnormal baseline blood chemistry (such as low albumin)

How to Handle Common Objections to MMT

My doctor says diet doesn't matter.

Many physicians have never received any substantive training on nutrition, which can result in them being skeptical about the value of making dietary changes to treat or prevent disease. Take this objection as merely an indication of a fatal flaw in our medical education system, and not as a personal prognosis of success or failure. If they believe that diet truly doesn't matter, then they should also believe that it won't hurt if you alter the way you eat.

There's no concrete evidence that a fat-burning diet has a therapeutic effect on disease.

At this time the only scientific proof that a high-fat, low-carb diet has a beneficial effect relates to children with drug-resistant seizures. However this does not mean that it doesn't work for other conditions, only that the trials needed to show an effect are still many years out and will require loads of funding that is not typically dedicated to diet studies. Please understand that there are no studies that show it does not work. Review Chapter 2 for a comprehensive list of recent and important studies on the effects of high-fat diets on disease.

My doctor doesn't want me eating this much fat.

The current government dietary guidelines limit calories from fat to around 20 to 35 percent of your total. These guidelines are based on flawed science, yet they persist. Fortunately, in recent years some bright and dedicated researchers have started to unravel these myths. What they're learning is that excess carbohydrates, especially the easily digestible ones from grains, starches, and fruits, are the primary cause of many of the chronic diseases that degrade health from childhood on.

This eating plan is too restrictive and hard to implement. I don't want to weigh everything.

It may seem tedious to weigh your food, record your food intake, and test your glucose levels—I'm not going to pretend it's not. But you don't have to start out keeping meticulous records. You can begin at whatever level of tracking and testing is doable for you, and gradually increase your record keeping over time, as other parts of the plan become easier.

Also, take a moment to consider how inconvenient, expensive, and unpleasant the conventional therapies can be: chemo, radiation, surgery, and dangerous—potentially life-threatening—medications are terribly inconvenient, as are frustration over not being able to lose weight and a sense of disempowerment regarding your own body and health. While MMT is not a cure, it is a powerful foundational metabolic intervention that will kick-start your body to begin the healing process. Of course this requires more effort on your part, and you need commitment to put your plan into action. But the upside far outweighs the minor inconvenience of weighing your portions and keeping good records of your progress.

I need a complete meal plan in order to do this.

Miriam Kalamian, the nutritionist who specializes in helping clients who have cancer adopt a fat-burning diet and who has consulted extensively on this book, hears this a lot but knows that in reality, you can start very simply. That's why she and I collaborated on three different ways to embark on MMT, which we call "on-ramps" and which we cover in the next chapter. While you may believe you need each meal mapped out for you in advance, you actually only need to think of your new plan one meal at a time. If you are feeling overwhelmed just thinking about these changes, start with one high-fat meal per day and you'll find it easier to quickly work your way up to a full day of fat-burning meals.

There are plenty of websites, cookbooks, and even meal-planning services that you can use as resources to help you draw up a detailed and personalized meal plan. But you don't need a plan like this to get started. In fact, the more you personally engage in the research and decision making, the more able you'll be to make MMT work for you and your particular health situation.

If you still feel like there are too many obstacles to making these changes, consider working with a health coach or nutritionist who specializes in therapeutic high-fat diets (see page 192 for info on how to find one). Most likely, all you really need is a few hours of consultation to create your personal road map.

My doctor doesn't want me to lose weight.

If you are at or above a healthy weight, losing a little weight can work to heal some of the underlying conditions of disease, such as insulin resistance. That said, I understand that your doctor may not want you to lose weight, particularly if you have cancer (as unintended weight loss can be a sign that you are not tolerating the standard treatments well, or that your disease is progressing). If you are already underweight, you can set up your high-fat eating plan to provide more calories than are required to maintain your current weight so you gain weight on the plan.

I can't afford organic/I can't find high-quality foods locally.

That's okay. It's better to work within these limitations than to let them keep you from making any beneficial changes. Work to the best of your ability dependent on where you are right now in terms of health, cooking ability, budget, and food availability. The important element here is to make the commitment to start. Once you've experienced the benefits for yourself—for example, seen your blood sugar drop to a new and healthier level—you will be motivated to find ways to improve on the quality of the foods in your plan.

I don't have the time for shopping and meal prep.

This is another challenge that Miriam runs up against frequently. Her advice: Chances are you're already spending some time in the grocery store and the kitchen. Find some easy-to-prepare, high-fat, low-carbohydrate recipes online that you think you might enjoy and then check to see if you have all the ingredients. If not, add them to your shopping list. (Yes, you'll need a shopping list as you'll be visiting different areas of the supermarket.) Another option: ask your friends or family to help you out here. You may not get exactly what you want on the first try but it's a step in the right direction.

I need to keep non-MMT foods on hand for my kids (or spouse).

The reality is that these foods are no better for your family members than they are for you. While you can't force others to adopt MMT, you can set a good example by switching to a fat-burning diet; use this as an opportunity to improve your entire family's health. Plus, your kids and/or spouse will still have plenty of access to these foods outside the home—no need to keep your cupboards and fridge stocked with all manner of carb- and sugar-laden treats.

If there are some foods that are high in quality but aren't part of the fat-burning food plan, especially if they are appropriate choices for the youngest members of your family, designate a clear "Non-MMT" area to store them in. Then accept as fact that these areas are off limits to you.

My doctor/friend says I'll get kidney stones.

MMT changes the way your kidneys handle sodium, which can result in a loss of both sodium and water. The risk of kidney stones rises if you are not well hydrated because your urine will contain higher concentrations of substances—including calcium, oxalate, urate, cysteine, xanthine, and phosphate—that can precipitate out and form stones. Some foods on the fat-burning food plan are also high in oxalates, another possible contributor to the formation of some types of kidney stones. If you have a family or personal history of kidney stones, talk to your doctor about a prophylactic supplement—such as prescription potassium citrate. And everyone on MMT should stay well hydrated, drinking plenty of filtered tap water each day.

If you are working with a doctor who doesn't acknowledge your right to share in the decision making about your health, or who doesn't understand your perspective and concerns, start the search for a new doctor. Yes, you have incredible power over your health through your food choices, but you need a solid and supportive team, especially if you are facing a serious diagnosis. And every member of that team is important.

CHAPTER 7

HOW TO GET STARTED

At this point, we've covered the tools you will need and the tests you should have done before you adopt a fat-burning diet. Now it's time to review how to start making healthy food choices and creating the conditions for you to heal your mitochondrial metabolism.

Here are the steps to take to make your experience with MMT as successful as possible, right from the start.

STOCK YOUR KITCHEN WITH MMT-FRIENDLY FOODS

As soon as possible, get to the grocery store and buy plenty of MMT-friendly foods to stock the shelves of your cupboards and fridge. It's crucial that you do this *before* you start getting rid of carb- or sugar-laden foods, because you want to avoid that "I'm starving—what can I eat?" feeling that drives you to make poor choices.

Allow yourself plenty of time for shopping so you can carefully read labels and explore parts of the market that may be unfamiliar to you.

Refer back to Chapter 5 for a full discussion of the foods that are integral to MMT. I've also created a one-page shopping list you can refer to quickly when making your grocery list so you know which items should go into your cart. For extra credit, decide on two or three MMT-friendly recipes that appeal to you (see the sidebar on page 162 for good sources) and then be sure that the ingredients for these meals or snacks are on your shopping list.

Once you have several fat-burning foods in your refrigerator and on your pantry shelves, you can proceed with purging your pantry of any carb-, starch-, or sugar-laden foods. Following this order of tasks will help you feel supported during your transition to a new way of eating, and feeling supported will motivate you to keeping going. Let your benchmark be progress, not perfection.

MMT-Friendly Foods

Photocopy this list and take it with you to the grocery store on your first few shopping trips to help you restock your kitchen with foods that will ease your transition to fat burning.

Vegetables:

- Asparagus
- Avocados
- Broccoli
- Brussels sprouts
- Cabbage
- Cauliflower
- Celery
- Cucumbers
- Kale
- Mushrooms
- Salad greens

- Sauté greens
- Spinach
- Zucchini

After you are fat adapted, you can add back limited amounts of these foods:

- Eggplant
- Garlic
- Onions
- Parsnips
- Peppers
- Rutabaga
- Tomatoes
- Winter squash (very limited amounts)

Fruits:

- Berries (a small handful, in lieu of a serving of vegetables)
- Grapefruit (a few sections, replacing a serving of veggies)

Proteins:

- Grass-fed beef (ideally with the AGA American Grassfed certification)
- Lamb
- Pork (including limited amounts of bacon and sausage)
- Poultry (preferably pastured and organic)
- Seafood (wild-caught fish and shellfish)
- Sardines and anchovies
- Wild game meats
- Eggs (preferably pastured and organic)
- Organ meats

Dairy

- Cheese (hard cheeses such as cheddar or Parmesan or soft, high-fat cheese such as Brie)
- Heavy whipping cream
- Sour cream (cultured, without added starches or fillers)
- Full-fat "original" cream cheese

Nuts and Seeds

- Macadamias (rich in healthy fats, yet low in carbs and protein)
- Pecans
- Brazil nuts (rich in selenium but limit yourself to two per day because they are high in protein)
- Coconut (including unsweetened meat, milk, cream, or flour)
- Hazelnuts
- Chia seeds
- Hemp hearts/seeds
- Pumpkin seeds
- Black sesame seeds
- Black cumin seeds
- Raw cacao nibs
- Flax seeds (rich in healthy omega-3s and fiber; grind just before eating)

Snacks

- Avocados
- Olives
- Pickles (naturally fermented—look for salt on the ingredient list and no vinegar)

Fats and Oils

- Coconut oil

- MCT oil

- Cocoa butter

- Raw, organic butter or ghee, grass fed

- Lard or tallow from organically raised animals, best for sautéing

- Other saturated animal fats, such as duck fat

- Extra virgin olive oil (for dressings or homemade mayonnaise)

- Fermented vegetables, ideally made at home or bought (unpasteurized) and used as a condiment

Sweeteners

- Stevia (liquid drops, preferably organic)

- Lo han kuo or monk fruit

- Xylitol—although beware; it's toxic to dogs!

- Erythritol

REMOVE TEMPTATION WITH A PANTRY SWEEP

It is so much easier to resist the urge to eat carbs if they aren't in your home. An essential part of your preparation for adopting MMT is going through your pantry and cupboards and removing anything that is not compatible with the plan. Give it away to friends, or take it to a food bank. You may even be able to return unopened packaged foods to your grocery store and use the money you get back to purchase foods that are MMT friendly. The more quickly you work through this step, the less likely it is that you'll run into temptation.

LEARN TO READ LABELS

As you're doing your pantry sweep and evaluating new foods to bring into your home, it's important to upgrade your label reading skills so you can determine whether a food is appropriate for your fat-burning diet. Start with the most important line on any nutritional label: total carbohydrates. This is even more important than looking at the sugars because the sugar that makes up starch chains is often not listed on the label. Amazingly, the convoluted and confusing rules that govern what's called a sugar allows a free pass to starches that contain chains of glucose that are more than three molecules long. This sleight of hand won't escape detection by your body, though, and this glucose will ultimately circulate in your bloodstream in exactly the same way as the glucose in table sugar. So if the label says 0 grams of sugar and 20 grams of carbs, that food will not be appropriate for the MMT diet.

The second most important line to read is the fiber. Although fiber is a carb, the glucose molecules are bound in a way that can't end up in circulation so it doesn't have an impact on glucose or insulin. Bonus: fiber contributes to your overall health, in part by feeding your good gut bacteria. To determine net carbs, subtract the number of grams of fiber from the total grams of carbohydrates listed on the label. The one caveat that Miriam points out is if the food is highly processed and contains a lot of supplemental fiber—such as a low-carb tortilla—you want to subtract only half the number of fiber grams listed from the carbohydrate total, as some of that added fiber might be the type that can cause a rise in glucose or insulin. With few exceptions, this is not true with the fiber found in whole foods.

Returning to the label, you also want to make sure there are no hydrogenated fats listed in the ingredients. Through yet another loophole, manufacturers can include these health-destroying oils, but as long as the amount per serving is below 0.5 g, they can list the amount of trans fat as "0 grams." You want polyunsaturated fats to be low because polyunsaturated fats are omega-6s and most of those come from highly refined and inflammatory sources. It doesn't take much to tip the omega-6-to-omega-3 ratio in an unhealthy direction. Pay attention to the saturated fat line too, but know that saturated fats are welcome on the MMT plan, although they are typically demonized by all traditional nutritional advice.

Don't buy or eat a food unless you know and recognize each ingredient on the package.

Organic cane syrup, maple syrup, honey, and agave nectar are no more appropriate on this diet than table sugar. Look for the list of sneaky sugars included in the sidebar on page 150. They include ingredients like modified food starch. Even soy sauce can contribute small but significant amounts of carbs. Don't waste your allotment on these empty foods!

Get the Sugar out of Your Diet

Whether you have been eating a typical American diet, or even a whole foods–based diet, it is highly likely that more than half of the calories you've been consuming are derived from foods overloaded with carbs. And not just obvious sugars like those in sweet treats and desserts, but the glucose and other sugars that are contained in the starches, grains, fruits, dairy, and legumes you've been eating.

Remember that to train your body to burn fat for fuel, you have to dramatically reduce your intake of all forms of sugar. You will need to reduce your net carbs (total carbs minus fiber) to lower than 40 grams a day. It will take at least a few weeks to a few months before your body fully adapts to burning fat as your primary fuel.

You may be able to understand this concept intellectually, but it can be difficult to truly root out and remove all forms of sugar from your diet, for four main reasons:

1. **Your body is currently dependent on frequently replenished glucose.** When you stop eating foods that are ultimately converted to sugar in your body, before it has adapted to burning fat as its primary fuel, you will continue to experience hunger and cravings as

your glycogen stores get depleted and your liver isn't yet able to crank out ketones as an alternative cleaner fuel than glucose.

As Miriam describes it, "Eating carb-rich raises glucose, which then triggers the release of insulin. Then insulin pushes glucose out of the bloodstream, causing your blood sugar levels to drop. This change sends signals to your brain that you experience as hunger. It's a vicious cycle that you will have to push past. For some people, the cravings only last a couple of days, for others it's a week or more."

The good news is that once you have made the transition to fat burning, your cravings for sugar and starches, including junk foods, will evaporate as if by magic, and you will effortlessly go for hours between meals without experiencing the slightest pangs of hunger.

The even better news is that once you have shifted your body to burning fat as its primary fuel, you will regularly introduce several feasting days a month in which your net-carb intake can climb to 100 to 150 grams of net carbs per day. This will prevent your insulin levels from becoming too low.

2. **Without even knowing it, you have been eating foods that are made up primarily of sugars.** Even foods you thought were "safe" may be loaded with added sugars. (See the sidebar on page 150 for Surprising Sources of Hidden Sugars.) As a result, you will likely have moments of wondering, "What exactly *can* I eat?"

   Keep referring back to your list of MMT-friendly foods (on pages 142–145) and make sure you have those foods on hand. I find that a handful of macadamia nuts or pecans stave off hunger quite nicely and are easy to bring with me wherever I go. Find a couple of go-to foods and make sure you have access to

them at work, in your car, and at home so you aren't
tempted to grab a bag of chips.

3.   **It can be challenging to eat enough calories from fat
     to adequately replace the calories you were getting
     from sugars and starches, especially in the begin-
     ning of adopting a fat-burning diet.** People have been
     trained to avoid eating fats. It doesn't come naturally
     at first, so chances are you won't be replacing all the
     calories you're taking out. That puts you at a deficit,
     which can only intensify hunger until you've made
     the transition to burning fat. Entering all your foods in
     Cronometer in real time will help you see this for your-
     self so you can address the problem quickly.

     The good news is that once you have made the
     transition, you will effortlessly go 13 to 18 hours with-
     out the need to eat during your daily fast because you
     will be burning fat stores for fuel so your body won't
     be sending out hunger signals. During the transition,
     fat bombs, avocados, and macadamia nuts come in
     very handy, as they are tasty and convenient ways to
     consume a tablespoon—or more—of healthy fats to
     fill in that energy gap.

4.   **Your cravings may be a need for emotional support.**
     If you've been eating carb-rich foods for comfort, your
     cravings are emotional as well as physical and will be
     more of a challenge to overcome. Eating a fat bomb
     might replace the brownie you would have otherwise
     eaten, but if you were relying on that food for comfort,
     your challenge is to find a new way to feel loved and
     cared for. Your support network, including caregivers,
     can play an important role here. Also, one of my favor-
     ite ways to address emotional issues is the Emotional
     Freedom Technique—a DIY form of acupressure that
     releases stuck emotions and helps reframe old beliefs.
     Visit eft.mercola.com to learn more.

Surprising Sources of Hidden Sugars

Condiments	Beverages	Snacks	Meals
Salsa	Lattes	Fresh or dried fruit	Many Thai and Vietnamese dishes, such as pad Thai
Ketchup	Flavored coffees	Flavored yogurt	Frozen dinners
Packaged salad dressings	Iced tea beverages	Peanut butter with added sugars	
Barbecue sauce	Flavored kefir	Nut butters with added sugars	
Teriyaki sauce	Commercially prepared smoothies		
Bottled marinades	Most mixed drinks		
Pickles	Sweet white and sparkling wines		
Relish	Creamers, dairy or nondairy		
Honey mustard	Dairy-free milks (look for the word "unsweetened" on the box)		
Commercially prepared coleslaw	Juices that contain fruits and root vegetables		
Tomato sauce			

It's Better to Go Cold Turkey on the Sugar Purge

I know there are many occasions where it will be tempting to have "just a bite" of a cake or dessert—a child's birthday party, a family celebration, or even dining out at a fine restaurant. But eating any sugar is setting yourself on a slippery slope. Sugar is addictive and not easy to resist using willpower alone. Also, eating a few too many carbs here and there will make it harder for you to transition to full fat burning, which interferes with the elimination of your cravings for sugar.

Also, you're not likely to be successful with the plan if you're willing to make exceptions—there's just not that much leeway in MMT, particularly in the beginning when you are trying to train your body to burn fat. The best way to stay committed to your plan is to build new traditions that don't revolve around food.

For a variety of reasons, you may want to hold on to some traditions, such as Thanksgiving dinner, so challenge yourself to find a great low-carb dish to bring to the table. Your friends and family might view your plan differently if they see that your foods are just as tasty as the standard offerings. Plan ahead by doing a quick Internet search using search terms like "ketogenic coconut custard" or "zucchini noodles." There are great recipes out there already and new ones are added daily. Your social occasions will be much more enjoyable if you are fully adapted to burn fat as your primary fuel. If the foods there will be a challenge, be sure to consume most of your food for the day before you leave home and you will sidestep cravings, helping you resist any unhealthy temptations.

Remember: you can't live in both worlds. If you continue to eat carbs and attempt to combine that with high fat, you will remain under the control of insulin signaling and that combination is dangerous to your health. Working with a health coach can go a long way toward finding ways to navigate the temptation to sneak in carbs here and there.

Determine Your Macronutrients

As I have mentioned, MMT is a high-fat, low-carb, and adequate-protein diet, and I covered the specific foods within each of these broader categories that are included on MMT in Chapter 5. Now it's time to drill down a little deeper and choose exactly how many grams of each of these macronutrients you'll consume on *your* version of MMT. By taking the time to calculate some specific targets, you'll have some invaluable guidelines to follow as you transition to burning fat.

I say "your version of MMT" because there is no one-size-fits-all answer to exactly how much of each macronutrient you should eat each day. These numbers need to be customized to your body and your state of health. Here's how to do that:

Protein

This is one of the key differentiating aspects of the MMT program. Unlike Atkins and most Paleo recommendations, MMT provides very precise protein recommendations to minimize the impact of activating mTOR and other biochemical signaling pathways and restore health to your mitochondria.

The general rule of thumb for determining how much protein to eat each day is to follow the formula of 1 gram of protein for every kilogram of lean body mass. To determine that number, you will first need to calculate your lean body mass. The simplest and easiest way is to compare yourself to pictures of people with varying body fat percentages. Although this is not precise, it is better than guessing or not entering any estimate at all (see Chapter 6 for information on the different assessment tools).

Once you have your body fat percentage, convert your weight in pounds into kilograms. Simply divide your weight in pounds by 2.2 to arrive at kilograms or use an online calculator (type "pounds to kilograms" into a Google search). Then multiply your weight in kilograms by your body fat percentage—that total is how much fat you're carrying in kilograms. Subtract that number from your total body weight to determine your lean body mass. Then multiply that number by 1.0 to get the number of grams of protein you should aim to eat in a day.

For example, for a 146-pound woman with 33 percent body fat (a typical amount for women at this weight):

146 pounds equals 66.22 kilograms

66.22 x .33 equals 21.85 kilograms of fat

66.22 - 21.85 equals 44.4 kilograms lean body mass

44.4 x 1 equals 44.4 grams of protein

In this example, 44 grams of protein divided over three meals means nearly 15 grams at each meal. For meat servings, a portion equal to ¼ of the size of a deck of cards contains 5 to 7 grams of protein. For fish, each ¼ of a checkbook-sized portion contains 5 to 7 grams. There is also some protein in vegetables, nuts, and seeds.

So, to get 15 grams of protein at lunch, this woman's meat serving should be about ½ to ¾ the size of a deck of cards.

Once you've determined the number of protein grams you'll need, it's helpful to start teaching yourself some visual cues for making sure that your portion sizes keep you on target. Weighing your portions and then entering them into Cronometer will help you train your eye to assess the proper portion size for each type of protein food you eat and give you very precise feedback on how much protein you're consuming. Being able to visualize portion sizes will also simplify eating out and make occasional travel less likely to derail your fat-burning food plan.

Again, MMT is highly individualized. If you have a serious illness, such as cancer, you may need to lower your intake of protein to minimize activity in the pathways that can contribute to disease. Work with a knowledgeable health coach or nutrition professional to help you determine what protein target is right for you, and understand that your needs may change over time.

Carbs

A guiding principle of MMT is to limit your intake of net carbs to under 50 grams per day, or 4 to 10 percent of your daily calories. Keep in mind that this number varies widely between individuals. The exact number of carbs that works best to keep your body in a fat-burning state may be much lower, especially if you're insulin resistant, mostly sedentary, or have type 2 diabetes. Then your upper limit may be as low as 20 grams, at least at the start of the plan.

Some people will need to keep their net-carb intake very low, 10 to 15 grams a day, to enter and stay in the fat-burning zone. Others will be able to go higher, to 40 grams or more. Even when you find the amount that works for you now, you may need to either tighten or loosen that over time, based on your health or goals and the feedback your body is providing you.

A good way to find a starting target is to consider these guidelines that Miriam uses with her clients:

- If your diet is currently carb heavy, with lots of processed foods and sugars, or you are facing an aggressive cancer (such as brain cancer), start with a low target, between 10 and 15 grams. Paring it down to the minimum will help you focus on eliminating all nonessential carbs in your diet (such as ketchup or salsa, which contain natural and hidden sugars).

- If you are already eating a primarily whole-food, Paleo-like diet, even if you are addressing a serious health challenge such as cancer, aim for 20 net carbs per day. This is also a good place to start if you are taking thyroid medication or dealing with adrenal fatigue. Choosing wisely will allow for the most variety in low-net-carb vegetables, which are rich in nutrients and fiber.

- If your current diet is nutritionally sound and you are adopting a fat-burning food plan simply to maximize your health, you can also set your initial target at 20 grams of carbs per day. You may find that you can increase carbs to 40 grams over time without seeing a negative impact on your blood glucose, but it is typically better to start low.

Once you have switched your body over to burning fat as your primary fuel, you may be able to consume a bit more, from 40 to 80 grams of net carbs per day, or if you are an athlete with high energy needs, perhaps even as high as 100 grams. Take care here, though, as you want to stay in that fat-burning state. This is where monitoring glucose and ketones as you experiment with introducing more carbs will come in handy. If glucose trends upward and you drop out of nutritional ketosis—that is, if your blood levels of ketones fall below 0.5 mmol/L—you have exceeded your carbohydrate tolerance.

Also remember that the carbohydrates that you reintroduce should still come mainly from fibrous, low-net-carb vegetables with perhaps a bit more fruit or a small portion of legumes or root vegetables—not grains or added sugars.

Your metabolism and activity levels can vary from day to day or week to week, so be realistic about your target and test the impact of these changes by keeping an eye on your blood glucose and ketone levels. Whatever the actual number of net carbs you aim to eat each day, the bottom line is that your personal ideal number of net carbs is likely far less than what you are currently eating.

Once you have a target number of grams of carbs, remember: this is *net* carbs. To determine your net carbs merely subtract the grams of fiber from the total grams of carbohydrate. Cronometer makes this very easy for you and calculates to the tenth of a gram so you know precisely where you stand.

You will find that that carbs add up fast if you aren't thoughtful in your food choices. For example, if you keep using your favorite sugar-free creamer in your coffee, you could easily spend six grams of your precious allotment before you've even had breakfast.

To familiarize yourself with the carb content of nutrition-packed foods, do an Internet search for "low-carb fruits and vegetables." Look for those you like or are willing to try. You won't find many low-carb fruits, though, so for now be content with berries (always choose organic). Also, develop the habit of carefully reading nutrition labels. Keep lists of foods you like that are also low carb; these will come in very handy when you're shopping for groceries and planning meals.

One important point: the lower your carbs, the more likely it is that you will quickly transition to a fat-burning machine. That said, you will also initially be more prone to experience transition side effects such as nausea, fatigue, brain fog, and constipation. (See page 181 for more information on how to handle side effects.)

Fat

Now that you've set your targets for protein and carb consumption, the majority of your remaining daily caloric intake will be in the form of healthy fat. Remember: as I discussed in Chapter 1, you want to avoid all refined vegetable and nut oils. They are pro-inflammatory, and most commercial ones are contaminated with toxic herbicides and solvents. Focus on adding saturated fats (like those found in animal proteins and coconut oil) and monounsaturated fats (avocado and olive oil), with the only polyunsaturated fats in your diet coming from nuts and seeds (see Chapter 5 for a list and other information on nuts and seeds and remember that flax seeds need to be ground before you eat them to improve the bioavailability of their nutrients).

Also remember that you do not want to consume more than 3 to 4 percent of your total calories as omega-6 fats because they will damage your cellular and mitochondrial membranes. And keep in mind that animal-based saturated fats are generally high in protein—be sure to count that so you will not exceed your target protein levels.

You want to aim for having 70 to 85 percent of your total daily calories come from healthy fats. In general, that means you are taking in two to three tablespoons of added fat at each meal, and one tablespoon in at least one snack. (Of course, this will vary one way or another according to your personal energy needs.) Although this guideline is simple, eating this much fat is so far outside the boundaries of what you've been taught that, once you pull out the excess carbs and protein, it can be hard to take in enough calories unless you get into the habit of eating more fat. Give your palate and your mind time to adjust to eating this much fat at every meal.

This is clearly a high-fat diet and many people simply can't properly break fats down. This is especially true if you have had your gallbladder removed. If you fall into this category, it is imperative that you take two supplements—ox bile and a digestive enzyme with plenty of the enzyme lipase. Take these every time you eat a high-fat food, and they should radically improve your ability to digest healthy fats.

To help increase your daily fat intake, go online and find recipes for simple fat bombs (a quick web search will provide hundreds of options). Having these on hand can make your early days of a fat-burning diet a lot more enjoyable. If you stick to it, you *will* transition to burning fat, and you will enjoy reduced hunger and a dramatic reduction in cravings for sweets. And if you are like most people, you have struggled with that your entire life.

CHOOSE YOUR STARTING POINT

I realize that I have referred to MMT as a "fat-burning diet." Although it *is* a comprehensive eating plan, MMT is less of a diet and more of a continuum of health and lifestyle improvements. It evolves, but it doesn't necessarily have an end (although, once you have been in fat-burning mode for a while, you should go through periods where you raise your net-carb intake, something I will explain in Chapter 10).

Since following a fat-burning food plan is a continuum, there are many ways to get started—I like to think of them as on-ramps. I've worked with Miriam to outline your three basic on-ramp options, the reasons why one might make more sense for you, and the particulars of what that course of action will look like in your daily life.

Multiple factors go into helping you decide which on-ramp is best for you. They include:

- **Your current diet.** Do you eat a primarily whole-foods, Paleo-type diet, or do you pretty much exist on packaged or prepared foods? The fat-burning food plan is less of a potential shock to your current palate if you are already eating a mostly healthy diet. For example, if you already prepare most of your meals at home, using whole foods, you may be able to dive right into a fat-burning plan. However, if you don't have much experience in the kitchen, a more gradual, stepped approach may make more sense for you.

- **Your current health.** Are you newly diagnosed? How extensive is your disease, and is there a risk that you will die from it in the near future? How resilient are you? Are you over- or underweight? If your health is already compromised by conventional therapies such as multiple rounds of chemotherapy, or if you are underweight, you will likely benefit from easing into the plan.

- **Your support network.** Are family and friends willing to help you with cooking, shopping, or emotional support? Or are you raising young kids, either on your own or while your spouse works? Are your loved ones supportive of your adopting a high-fat diet or are they skeptical? What about support from your physicians?

    You need confidence in order to stay committed, and occasionally you will need a boost of support to keep going. If you don't have strong support, you can still absolutely adopt this style of eating, but understand that you are more likely to be successful if you give yourself time and space to get organized first. Once you experience some of the early benefits, such as freedom from cravings and increased energy, that will naturally fuel your excitement and provide the motivation you need to keep going.

Working with a health coach who specializes in helping people make the transition to burning fat for fuel can be an extremely powerful way to boost your odds of success. Family members, friends, or other caregivers committed to helping you can also serve as coaches if they are willing to do the research that will help you wisely choose the on-ramp best suited to your health and current diet. At the very least, call on your team to help you gather supplies, shop for the right foods, and prepare delicious meals.

There's no one right way to get started. The right choice is the course of action that helps you make steady progress. Meaning, how you start doesn't matter as much as how you move along the continuum, so choose what feels like the best match for you at this time.

On-Ramp #1: Ease In

Pros: Gives you a chance to get organized by slowly purging your pantry, shopping for new ingredients, and researching a couple of recipes that you'll use in the beginning. Prevents feeling overwhelmed by giving you a chance to test meals and master each new skill before moving on the next. It also allows you to gradually adjust your palate and switch your food-prep habits to include more high-fat foods in your meals.

Easing in also helps you avoid the side effects of rapid weight loss, which can include the release of a surge of hormones and toxins, previously stored in the fat cells, into the bloodstream all at once. It can also reduce a set of symptoms commonly referred to as the "keto flu" that include nausea, fatigue, muscle aches, and brain fog, which can occur as your body switches from one primary fuel to another.

Cons: The only major disadvantage of this approach is that you could lose precious time if you have a serious illness that is causing a rapid deterioration. But if that is not your challenge, a gradual start to MMT may even have some advantages over diving in or jump-starting with a fast: a 2005 randomized prospective study found that children with seizures who were assigned to a gradual start of a fat-burning food plan had fewer side effects and better tolerance than children who started the diet with a fast.[1]

How to do it: Start with one high-fat, moderate-protein, low-carbohydrate meal a day. Miriam suggests breakfast: two eggs cooked in one tablespoon of butter or ghee and one tablespoon coconut oil. The eggs will absorb the oils and won't feel overly greasy. Be sure that you are also working through the "Getting Started Checklist" (see page 172).

Enter this breakfast into Cronometer so you can view the important feedback regarding your nutrient intake.

As your breakfast routine becomes well established, you can move to eating high fat at lunch too. Have a salad consisting of several cups of leafy greens, half to a whole avocado, some form of protein (portion size will depend on your daily protein needs, which I covered earlier in this chapter). Include other low-carb vegetables (such as broccoli or zucchini) drizzled with pastured butter. Miriam believes it's okay to sprinkle some grated cheese over the top of the salad too, so long as you keep it to a condiment-sized portion and count it as part of your day's food intake.

Enter all ingredients, with their weight in grams, into Cronometer. If you use the same basic salad ingredients every day, you can save time in the long run by entering these as one recipe. You can then add the protein food separately, depending on your choice for that day.

Next, move to making dinner a high-fat meal as well. If needed, add in some high-fat snacks between lunch and dinner until you are eating high fat all the time. At the same time, you'll be pulling away from the high net carbs that made up a large part of your former way of eating.

Feel free to experiment with a variety of high-fat recipes. As you add more high-fat foods into your regular rotation, start entering your favorite combinations into Cronometer as full recipes so that later, when you are eating high fat all the time, it's almost effortless to record your most common choices.

Sample One-Day Eating Plan for the "Ease In" On-Ramp

- As You Start Your Day
  Measure your glucose level when you first wake up. If you aren't hungry yet, don't eat anything. Wait until you're truly hungry.

- Breakfast
  Time: When your hunger becomes noticeable.
  What: Mostly protein and fats, such as two eggs cooked in one tablespoon ghee and one tablespoon coconut oil, or one egg with two strips of bacon (to keep your protein intake adequate but not excessive). If you need something faster, try a smoothie made out of unsweetened almond milk, unsweetened protein powder (check the carbs on the label), cream, a tablespoon of coconut milk or a teaspoon of MCT oil, two strawberries or a small handful of blueberries, and stevia to taste.

- Lunch
  Time: A few hours after your first meal.
  What: A typical lunch for you, although you're aiming to reduce the number of carbs. If you usually have a sandwich, make it open faced. If you usually have a bowl of pasta, get a hearty soup instead.

- Dinner
  Time: Start to eat dinner a little earlier than you usually do—perhaps as long as three hours before bedtime, but any change here is good.
  What: Eat a normal dinner for you, but include more low-net-carb vegetables than you would normally eat and a smaller protein serving than you would normally eat.

- Snacks

  Time: As needed.

  What: A handful of macadamia nuts, or a tablespoon of almond butter mixed with a teaspoon of coconut oil spread on a celery stick.

- Before Bed

  Test and record your glucose level so you can track how it trends over time.

Good Online Sources of High-Fat, Low-Carb, Moderate-Protein Recipes

www.ketodietapp.com (search for "60 amazing fat bombs")

www.ruled.me

www.ketogenic-diet-resource.com

www.charliefoundation.org

You can also search online using the keyword "keto." Don't use "low carb" or "high fat," as it will often yield recipes that are too high in protein.

On-Ramp #2: Dive In

Pros: You may be highly motivated to start eating differently and improving your mitochondrial metabolism, and this approach lets you get your feet wet while making progress right away. This is also a useful strategy if you have a serious health challenge that requires immediate intervention.

Cons: You may feel overwhelmed if you attempt to dive in before you've stocked your refrigerator and pantry with the right foods. You may also experience more side effects as you make the switch to burning fat as fuel, including nausea, brain fog, fatigue, and muscle cramping. Also, if you dive in you are more likely to experience rapid weight loss, which may or may not be desirable based on your current weight and health status.

How to do it: Reduce your net carbs to between 20 and 25 grams a day, limit your protein to 1 gram/kilogram of lean body mass (see page 152 for more information on setting your carb and protein targets), and replace a significant part of those calories with high-quality fat sources. *You will really have to challenge yourself to consume enough fat in the beginning.* Depending on your calorie requirements, you may need to add the equivalent of three or more tablespoons of fat with each of your three main meals, and one or more tablespoons in your snack.

In addition, you'll want to consume these meals within a compressed eating window, as I discuss in Chapter 10. It's also very important to mitochondrial health to stop eating at least three hours before bedtime, allowing for a 13- to 18-hour window before the next time you take a bite of food. (For example, if your last meal is at 5 P.M., your first meal the next day might be at 9 A.M.)

Start by keeping your meals very simple—see the sidebar for a guideline on meal planning.

Begin tracking your blood glucose levels using your home glucose monitor (described in Chapter 6). Test three times a day according to this schedule:

- When you first wake up (before you've had anything to eat or drink, including coffee or tea). This is your fasting blood glucose.

- Right before you eat your first meal of the day. In an ideal situation, you'd wait to eat until your blood glucose level is below 80 (although many people may never get readings this low due to a preexisting health condition).

- At bedtime. This reading gives you feedback on your food choices for that day.

Many glucose monitors will store your previous readings, but I recommend recording your results, ideally in Cronometer. As you first embark on the diet and your body makes the transition to fat burning, you will likely get readings that jump from high to low. But as your body gradually learns how to burn fat as your primary fuel, you will see your numbers stabilize and trend downward over time. This is incredibly empowering and will give you a strong sense of gratification along with the motivation to stay committed to your new plan.

Start tracking your food intake at Cronometer.com/mercola. Start with one meal a day and work your way up to recording everything you eat. If you spend some time entering your most frequent meals as recipes, you will find that entering your daily foods takes only a few minutes a day. The program will not only help you see your progress, but also easily allow you to share your food record and nutrient profile with your health care professional or coach. (Remember: if tracking is too overwhelming for you, you can plan what you eat instead, using Cronometer to check nutrient values.)

Setting up your profile and entering some specific meals that you plan to use often will take a few hours of your time. But after that initial effort, it will only require a few minutes a day to enter your foods and track your data.

Sample One-Day Eating Plan for the "Dive In" On-Ramp

- As You Start Your Day

  Measure your glucose level before you eat or drink anything. Then enjoy your coffee or tea with one to two tablespoons of grass-fed butter, coconut oil, or MCT oil melted into it. Optional: froth it with an immersion blender.

- Breakfast

  Time: Delay this first meal until you feel truly hungry. As I will discuss in Chapter 10, extending the periods of time you go without food has many metabolic benefits. Over time, you'll work up to going 13 to 18 hours between your last meal of the previous day and your first meal of this new day.

  What: predominately protein and fats. Examples: eggs cooked in one tablespoon of ghee and one tablespoon of coconut oil. Optional: add in shredded zucchini or spinach.

Or enjoy a coconut milk smoothie with half of an avocado, a tablespoon or two of heavy cream or coconut oil to boost the fat, and about one ounce of a mixture of freshly ground seeds. Add stevia as needed.

- Lunch

    Time: ideally, when your glucose reading is 80 or lower, or a few hours after your first meal.

    What: two to three cups of salad greens, half an avocado, an appropriate-for-you-sized portion of protein (such as chicken, fish or lamb—use your scale for precise measurement), two tablespoons extra virgin olive oil, a splash of white wine vinegar, and (optional) two tablespoons of a hard cheese (such as Parmesan) grated over the top.

- Dinner

    Time: at least three hours before bedtime, as eating at night, when your energy needs are low, can flood your mitochondria with ROS. I will discuss this more in Chapter 10, but for now, aim to eat dinner a little earlier than you typically do.

    What: start with a right-for-you portion of protein such as salmon, beef, or chicken, cooked in plenty of high-quality fat— duck fat, bacon grease, lard, or ghee—plus a low-carb veggie served with plenty of butter or olive oil or coconut oil. Ideally, this should be a lighter meal than breakfast and lunch. Remember: you will generate more unwanted free radicals if you eat large amounts of fuel just before sleep, at a time when you need them the least. It will also result in mitochondrial damage because it prevents the overnight housekeeping activities that contribute to cellular health.

- Snacks:

    Time: as needed during your eating window.

    What: macadamia nuts, pecans, celery, avocado, fat bombs.

On-Ramp #3: Jump-Start with a Water Fast

If you are basically healthy or don't have weight to lose, I believe this is not the best strategy because it will clearly result in weight loss. If, like the majority of the population, you are overweight, this may be the best choice as it will help jump-start your body's ability to burn fat as your primary fuel. So rather than taking a few months or longer to achieve fat-burning capability, you might be able to achieve this state after a few rounds of a few days of fasting (see Chapter 10 for more details on how to fast).

The time you save in food shopping and preparation you can put toward a pantry sweep (discussed earlier in this chapter), removing unhealthy foods from your home and replacing them with those that are more aligned with helping you succeed in burning fat as your primary fuel.

Sample Water Fast Protocol

A water fast isn't limited to just water—there are other fluids (and even some seeds) allowed. Here's your guide to what you can use to stay hydrated and derive some nutrients while giving your digestion a rest and your body a chance to jump-start fat burning:

Fluids allowed:

- Water (unlimited)

- Tea (unlimited)

- Coffee (up to six cups a day, hot or iced)

- Homemade broth (unlimited, although you'll notice that you need less as you become more acclimated to fasting)

What you can add to your water:

- Lime slices (don't consume the limes or any other fruits)

- Lemon slices

- Apple cider vinegar (raw, organic, with "the mother," or the culture of beneficial bacteria that converted regular apple cider into vinegar)

- Himalayan salt

What you can add to your coffee or tea (up to one tablespoon):

- Coconut oil
- MCT oil
- Butter (organic, pastured, preferably raw)
- Ghee (organic, pastured, preferably raw)
- Heavy cream (organic, pastured, preferably raw)
- Ground cinnamon
- Lemon (for tea)

What you can add to your broth as it cooks (strain before eating):

- Himalayan salt
- Any vegetable that grows above ground, particularly leafy greens
- Onions or shallots
- Carrots, chopped
- Animal bones
- Fish bones
- Any herbs and spices
- Whole organic flax seeds (one tablespoon per cup of broth)

Tips for a Successful Start

- **Have a plan for hunger.** In the first few days or weeks of the transition to fat burning, you may experience hunger, especially if you're not replacing carb calories with fat calories. Adding MCT oil to your food or drink will help fill the energy gap (refer back to Chapter 5 for more information on MCT oil). Just be careful to start with a small and tolerable amount, such as a teaspoon or two, and gradually build up to a tablespoon or more. Back off a bit if you begin to experience bloating or loose stools. If you don't tolerate much MCT (this varies widely), you can use coconut oil. Miriam suggests mixing a teaspoon or two into a tablespoon of almond butter and eating it on a celery stick, or you can swirl it into a cup of coffee or tea. Avocado is another great food to have on hand in these early days—you can eat it right out of the shell, sprinkled with sea salt and perhaps even drizzled with a little olive oil and a squeeze of fresh lemon. I promise you: you won't be hungry for long after snacking on an avocado! The fiber it contains makes it a very filling food, and it is high in potassium and monounsaturated fat.

- **Gather high-fat snacks to have on hand.** One of the most challenging parts of this plan is making sure you consume enough fat to keep you satiated and ward off cravings as your body transitions to burning fat. Make sure you are eating snacks that are *primarily fat* to manage hunger and energy in between your meals without boosting your intake of carbohydrates and protein. Here are some examples of high-fat snacks:

  - Fat bombs—small homemade candies or savory treats that contain a high percentage of fat, usually coconut oil; Google "fat bombs" for recipes

  - Avocados—eaten right out of the skin with a spoon and a sprinkle of sea salt, or mashed up as guacamole and eaten with a few pork rinds

  - Macadamia nuts, pecans, and Brazil nuts—macadamia nuts also make a great hummus. Caveat: limit Brazil nuts to two per day.

  - Coconut oil and/or butter and/or cream—mixed into coffee, tea, or a mug of broth

- Chia pudding—made with coconut milk and sweetened with stevia

- MCT oil—See Chapter 5 for guidelines on using this supplement

- **Add variety slowly.** In the first few days—or even weeks—of following the MMT eating plan, you will make things much easier on yourself if you stick to a handful of foods for your snacks and meals. This will make meal planning easier and will also allow you to see how these foods affect you and your glucose levels.

  As you get more comfortable with the basic points of a high-fat diet, you can begin to incorporate new recipes and food options. Remember: MMT is a continuum—there will always be new things to learn and recipes to try. Simply start at the level that makes the most sense for you, and refine from there.

- **Stay hydrated.** As you make the transition to burning fat, your kidneys will change the way they manage sodium levels, which results in your body releasing some of the water it's been holding on to. Along with that water will be some sodium and electrolytes, which may result in side effects such as muscle cramping, heart palpitations, or fatigue (I will cover side effects in Chapter 8). For this reason, be sure you are drinking plenty of filtered tap water in these early days of your high-fat eating plan, as well as adding natural Himalayan salt—which contains trace minerals and electrolytes—to your foods.

  Resist the urge to reach for sports drinks or even coconut water, as the sports drinks contain heaps of sugar or artificial sweeteners. Even coconut water contains a hefty dose of carbs.

Miriam's transition tip: if you experience any side effects, such as fatigue, brain fog, or muscle cramps, simply sipping on some homemade salted chicken, fish, or beef broth may be all you need to set yourself straight! Also, many new studies show that vitamin K_2 (as MK-7) will radically reduce nighttime muscle cramps, so it is best to take the K_2 before bedtime.

- **Find a way to record what you eat that works for you.** Personally, I love the precision of MMT, which includes weighing food, tracking intake, and testing glucose levels. But I realize there's a good chance that these elements may be intimidating or even over-whelming, especially in the first few weeks or months of the plan when so much may be new to you. Here, then, are a few reminders about why tracking your food intake and glucose levels is such a key piece of the fat-burning food plan:

  - *Real-time feedback so you can customize.* When you start tracking your food intake *and* your blood glucose levels, you will quickly learn how different foods and meals affect your numbers. This is crucial information that you can use to refine your plan as you keep moving forward toward your health goals. For example, you may come to see that caffeine causes a spike in your blood glucose levels. It's much better to know that caffeine is the culprit, rather than imagining other scenarios that make you question the efficacy of the diet. Or you may learn just the opposite: that a cup of coffee doesn't make a wrinkle in your day so there's no longer any reason to avoid it.

  - *Precision.* Unless you record every bit of food that passes your lips, you won't know for sure if the diet is having an effect on anything beyond weight loss. You need more data to see if you are making progress toward other goals—for example, lowering your fasting glucose. While I am offering guidelines for the plan in this book, you will still need to tailor it to your particular needs, health status, specific diagnosis, and goals. And you won't be able to make these refinements if you don't have clear data on what nutrients you are taking in and what nutrients you may still need.

- *Motivation.* When you can look at a list of everything you've eaten and track improvements in your glucose levels and other biometrics over time, it will motivate you to keep with the plan and continue refining it to meet your particular needs.

- *Commitment.* Staying with a fat-burning food plan absolutely requires commitment—there will be times, such as at family occasions or other social events, when sticking with it will be a challenge. Prepare for these inevitable situations and be open to ways you can learn from your mistakes.

- *Accountability.* As I mentioned, adopting a high-fat diet is an empowering choice. Tracking your food gives you a permanent record of your choices and helps you see how your actions create results in your body—both good and bad.

All that being said, if the idea of weighing your food, recording everything you eat in Cronometer, and monitoring your glucose levels multiple times a day are more than you are willing to take on right now, there is another option.

Instead of tracking your food consumption, you can plan it instead. Do this by following the Sample One-Day Eating Plan for the on-ramp you've chosen and simply write out what you will eat for the next day or few days, and then stick to that plan. Whether you are a planner or a tracker, you will have a record of all the food that you ate, so that you or your health coach

can see at a glance what your intake is relative to your
target allotments of carbs, protein, and fat. However,
this method will not give you as clear a picture as
tracking your overall nutrient intake, which is helpful
if you are trying to determine if you are getting enough
quantity, variety, and balance in your diet.

Getting Started Checklist

To help make this initial phase more manageable, Miriam and I
created this checklist so you can clearly see what you need to do:

_____ Start avoiding eating at least three hours before
bedtime.

_____ Start pushing the time of your first meal back to extend
the window of time between meals (experiment with adding
coconut oil and/or heavy cream to your morning coffee or tea to
make it easier to wait longer before eating).

_____ Get your preliminary blood work done (see pages
116–120).

_____ Purchase your glucose meter, glucose testing strips,
lancets, and keto strips if you choose to monitor your ketone
levels (see pages 110 and 115).

_____ Purchase a kitchen scale and candy molds (for making
fat bombs).

_____ Determine your macronutrient targets (see page 152).

_____ Make a copy of the MMT-friendly foods on pages 142–
145 to hang on your fridge and take with you to the grocery store.

_____ Buy MMT-friendly foods.

_____ Purge your pantry of foods not on the high-fat diet,
or clear out space in a cabinet designated specifically for MMT-
friendly foods.

_____ Begin testing your glucose levels three times a day—as
soon as you wake up, just before your first meal, and just before
bed—and tracking your results.

_____ Start eating as many high-fat, low-carb, moderate-
protein meals per day as matches the on-ramp you have chosen.

_____Open a Cronometer account and log your most frequently eaten meal.

_____Bookmark websites with recipes and information (see page 162).

_____Compile three to five recipes you want to start experimenting with.

_____As you get comfortable with each step of your new eating plan, keep refining it—seek out more recipes, log more of the food you eat, and do more research.

Clearing Long-Term Health Annoyances and Enjoying Renewed Energy

Jessica had a host of bizarre health issues, including recurring eczema, an inflamed eye, multiple allergies, hormonal issues, and struggles with weight loss. She had spent significant time and money on seeing physicians, but they had been able to offer her only marginal relief.

Jessica decided to consult with one more specialist before giving up, which is how she came to be in an office with Dr. Dan Pompa, a Salt Lake City health coach and cellular detox expert. To Dr. Pompa, Jessica's list of symptoms wasn't mysterious once he heard her health history.

Growing up, Jessica had been exposed to many toxins and molds and described herself as "a sick kid." As she had moved into her teens, she experienced depression, which intensified after her children were born. Her symptoms had been steadily piling up over a lifetime.

Dr. Pompa addressed her diet first. Jessica already leaned toward low carb and dabbled with higher fat because it made her feel better, but she had never felt confident that she was doing it right. With a few refinements to her existing diet, Jessica transitioned to fat burning right away. She then added daily intermittent fasting for five days a week, followed by one day of feasting and then one day of fasting.

In the beginning, Jessica would sometimes get off track. It helped that she kept tabs on her fasting blood glucose and ketones and also tested before meals. The feedback from this testing helped Jessica learn to pay attention to what her body *needed* instead of what she *wanted*.

For Jessica, putting all these elements together was magic. "The changes only took about five weeks. This was no time compared to all the years that I dealt with the bad stuff." (Frankly, oftentimes it takes longer so Dr. Pompa encourages patience.)

Although Jessica didn't lose many pounds overall, the inches melted off and she went down a couple of sizes. But the best effects had nothing to do with weight loss: "I have much more energy now and feel more purpose driven. My skin is clear and I feel healthy and very balanced in mind and body. Best of all, these are strategies I can continue for a lifetime."

CHAPTER 8

NAVIGATING YOUR TRANSITION TO BURNING FAT

Now that you've modified your diet to follow the fat-burning eating plan, your body will need to make the switch from burning glucose for fuel to burning fat. Be patient. This is a multistep process that can take anywhere from a few days to a few months, depending on your current health, your commitment to your macronutrient targets, and your metabolic flexibility as you begin to burn fat.

MMT is highly customizable to you and your body, and it may take a while to find the foods and practices that enable you to become fully fat adapted—I'll go into more detail on this in the next chapter. The aim of this chapter is to help you make the smoothest transition you can and get ahead of any possible challenges before they become big enough to potentially derail you.

What's Happening with Your Metabolism

Before you begin to burn fat, you must first use up the glycogen that is now stored in your skeletal muscles and your liver. In their book *The Art and Science of Low Carbohydrate Performance*, researchers Jeff Volek, Ph.D. and R.D., and Stephen Phinney, M.D. and Ph.D., estimate that glycogen stores in the average person top out at somewhere between 400 and 500 grams, of which 100 grams are stored in the liver. That translates to somewhere between 1,600 and 2,000 calories. If you have a lot of muscle mass and have eaten a high-carb diet, your stores may be higher than that.

Each gram of glycogen is stored with 3 to 4 grams of water, which means that as your stores are depleted, you will also lose this water weight, typically almost immediately after you begin restricting your carb intake. This is great news if one of your goals is weight loss.

As you can probably guess, burning 1,600 to 2,000 calories will only take a day or two—less time if you're active and more time if you're sedentary. But making the transition to burning fat isn't as simple as running through your glycogen. You also have to keep insulin levels low because insulin inhibits lipase, the hormone-sensitive enzyme that breaks down fat. Not only that, but you have to keep to this lower level for a couple of weeks to several months to fully activate your body's fat-burning system. Longer times are required for those who have profound insulin and leptin receptor resistance, especially if they are not using water fasts (covered as On-ramp #3 in Chapter 7 and again in more detail in Chapter 10).

Initially, your body will likely alternate between burning ketones, fatty acid, and glucose, which your liver can manufacture from excess protein, the breakdown of muscle tissue, or the freeing up of glycerol, which forms the backbone of triglycerides.

When you run out of glycogen, you may experience cravings for carbs and sweets, or feel hungry, because your body isn't particularly adept at burning fat for fuel yet. This temporary energy deficit may tempt you to sneak a few more carbs here and there, or to overeat protein, but this will backfire because it will keep you in this transition longer by supplying more glucose and more insulin. This will only delay the shift to burning fat.

As your glycogen stores become depleted, your liver takes on a larger role in maintaining a healthy level of blood glucose ("glucose homeostasis"). Before you started eating a high-fat diet, insulin and another pancreatic signaling hormone called glucagon were primarily responsible for tightly regulating your blood sugar levels. Now metabolic sensors in your liver are assuming that role, and they will at first seek to restore glycogen through the production of glucose, either from protein you've consumed or by breaking down skeletal muscle and/or using glycerol if you are consuming enough fat.

When your glucose levels are elevated, this will impair lipase from burning fat for fuel. It's only when you eliminate the interference of high glucose—either from dietary sources or from manufacture in the liver (gluconeogenesis)—that you begin to ramp up your fat burning. The longer and more consistently you restrict your intake of carbs while also limiting protein to 1 gram per kilogram of lean body mass or lower, the more efficient your liver will be as it figures out how to make this switch to burning fat for fuel.

The more compliant you are in the beginning of MMT, by really sticking to your macronutrient ratios and logging all the food you eat, the smoother this transition will be. Initially, even seemingly insignificant amounts of carbs will tend to cause a rise in your glucose, which will impair your fat burning. If you binge on carbs in the transition phase, you'll replenish your glycogen stores and lengthen the time it takes for you to shift to burning fat as your primary fuel.

As a general rule, the younger and healthier you are, the faster you can move through this transition. A school-age child can make the switch in 24 to 36 hours. While kids can transition much quicker, this does not mean they should be on this program unless they have intractable seizures or cancer.

Folks in their 20s and 30s have the easiest time of it, while people in their 40s and 50s will generally face a little more of a challenge (unless you are already fit and following a whole-foods,

Paleo-like diet). Those in their 60s and 70s will likely need to be very committed to make the switch. But if this is you, don't be discouraged; I started MMT at 61 and it only took a few weeks to shift to fat-burning mode.

If you are in your 80s or older, you can absolutely adopt the diet—it will likely just take a bit longer. Elderly individuals need to be monitored very carefully to prevent muscle loss (sarcopenia). The bottom line is that the sooner you get on board with MMT, the more easily you'll be able to sustain it and continue to enjoy the health benefits as you get older.

Use Your Blood Glucose Readings to Gauge Your Progress

Remember that you want to test your blood glucose levels two to three times a day: when you first wake up, just before you eat your first meal of the day, and just before you go to bed. During this transitional period, your glucose readings may show great variation, but erratic readings may be due to the fact that your meter is only a screening tool; just redo the test (see below). Even if the results are initially hard to interpret, as you continue with the eating plan you will see your readings settle down into a more predictable pattern.

Your blood glucose readings provide powerful feedback on how appropriate your food choices are: if your glucose numbers are high, it suggests that you've eaten too many net carbs and/or too much protein, although there can be other factors at work (see the sidebar on the next page for those).

While you will likely see spikes and dips in the beginning, you will get more adept at choosing foods that keep you in the fat-burning zone, and you will start to see your early-morning and late-night readings smoothing out over time. Even then, expect the occasional spike. Just remember: your focus is on the trend over the course of several days, or even weeks, and your reward is watching your glucose numbers go down and become more stable. That means your insulin isn't working as hard either.

Reasons Why You May Be Getting a High Glucose Reading

It can be alarming to measure your blood glucose levels and see some unexpectedly high readings. Here are some common triggers that may explain them:

- **Menstrual Hormones:** Glucose readings tend to be higher in the days just before the start of a woman's cycle.

- **Inflammation:** Injury, surgery, or illness can all lead to inflammation, which also causes a rise in blood sugar.

- **Too Much Protein:** Eating more than adequate protein throughout the day or at a particular meal can trigger the liver to manufacture new glucose through the process of gluconeogenesis.

- **Equipment Limitations:** Home blood glucose meters can be off as much as 20 percent in either direction. If you get an unusual or unexpected reading, immediately do another glucose test, using the same finger but a different blood drop. If you get a significantly different reading, do a third test, and take the average of all three.

- **Noncompliance:** Seemingly insignificant amounts of net carbs can disrupt your blood glucose levels. You may not even realize that your food choices have sugar in them, so if you are getting higher readings than you expect, look back on the food you've eaten in the last couple of hours. This includes reading labels.

- **Illness:** A cold, the flu, and seasonal allergies all stimulate the immune system, resulting in a natural rise in steroid hormone—and one of steroid's effects is to increase glucose levels.

- **Exercise:** If you have exercised vigorously in the hours prior to a high reading, it can mean that you ran out of ketones or you haven't made the shift to making ketones yet, triggering your body to break down muscle and convert it to glucose for fuel. Non-intense and gentle exercises like walking and yoga actually tend to lower glucose levels.

- **Stress:** Don't underestimate the impact of stress on blood glucose levels. When you experience real or imagined stress, you are likely to release adrenaline and cortisol, which trigger the manufacture of glucose.

- **Poor Sleep:** Each morning, your circadian rhythm prompts a release of cortisol to help you wake up, and cortisol triggers the release of glucose. After a night of too little sleep, your circadian rhythm and hormone balance are disrupted, which can lead to a surge in blood glucose levels.

- **Chemo and Radiation:** These treatments trigger inflammation that causes a rise in blood glucose—but you can take comfort in the fact that if you weren't doing the diet, your blood glucose would be a lot higher.

WHEN YOU EAT MATTERS

A way to enhance your transition to fat burning is to begin to experiment with regular periods of fasting. There are many ways to do this, and many powerful benefits to reap, all of which I cover in Chapter 10. For the time being, aim to finish your last meal at least three hours before bedtime, and then wait as long as possible before eating breakfast the next day. This will help you ease into my favorite form of intermittent fasting, which I call Peak Fasting.

THE SIZE OF YOUR MEAL MATTERS

Ideally, it is best to time your biggest meal for *before* your most active period of the day so your muscles—which remain responsive to glucose even when you're fat burning—will remove most of the extra glucose and insulin from your blood before they have the chance to disrupt your new fat-burning metabolism. Also ideally, you'd divide this largest meal in half and eat the second half 60 to 90 minutes after the first half, as this results in less nitrogen stress on your kidneys.

You also want to spread your protein consumption out over the day, limiting your protein at a given meal to about 15 grams. This makes it less likely that an excess of amino acids from protein will be converted into glucose by the liver, and it will also ease the detoxification burden on your kidneys. This is especially important if you already have some kidney insufficiency, with a serum creatinine level above 1. If this sounds like a low intake of protein to you, remember that excess amino acids are also a powerful stimulus to activate mTOR. (If you'd like a refresher on this information, refer back to Chapter 3.)

Especially during this transitional period, plan on having at least one or two high-fat snacks during the day. This will help tamp down any hunger or cravings and keep you feeling full and satisfied. (See the sidebar on page 144 for several high-fat snack suggestions.)

COMMON SYMPTOMS EXPERIENCED DURING THE TRANSITION TO FAT BURNING AND THEIR REMEDIES

As you make the switch to burning fat and your body relearns how to burn fat instead of glucose for fuel, it is normal to go through a period where you experience one or a couple of common symptoms. You can manage the intensity of these symptoms by deciding how quickly you'll change your diet, but you can't totally avoid all of them: your body is learning a new way to fuel itself, so expect a glitch or two as it finds its way.

Here are the most common symptoms and simple ways to ward them off:

- **Dehydration:** As you transition to burning fat, your kidneys will start handling sodium differently. This will encourage your body to release more water and with it, some electrolytes as well. Make sure you are drinking water throughout the day. Miriam counsels her patients to also sip on homemade chicken, fish, or beef broth that has been salted with Himalayan salt, as it will replace electrolytes you may lose. (That said, keep your broth consumption to a cup or so as it contains amino acids that can be converted to glucose in the liver.)

- **Nausea:** If you look at a fatty food and feel nauseated, adding a supplement high in the fat-digesting enzyme lipase can help you break down fats more easily. Look for a supplement with pancreatin, which contains lipase. Ox bile is another supplement that will help emulsify the fat and allow you to better absorb it.

- **Brain fog:** Your brain can't oxidize fatty acids for fuel but it will begin to use ketones for energy right away. In the early days, ketones only meet about a quarter of the brain's required fuel; for the rest of its energy needs, your brain will still be dependent on glucose. Over time, your brain will transition to deriving more of its energy—as much as 60 to 70 percent in some people—from ketones. So any brain fog you may experience initially is going to get better over time as your brain adjusts to using ketones for energy. Again, taking a little more coconut oil or MCT oil (to the level that your digestion can accommodate without stomach upset) can help.

- **Muscle cramps:** This is a very common symptom related to a change in electrolyte balance that is part of the normal switch to fat burning. You can restore some electrolytes by increasing your salt intake with ½ to 1 teaspoon of a healthy salt like Himalayan salt. Another option: take an Epsom salt bath—Epsom salts contain magnesium, a natural muscle relaxant that you can absorb transdermally. (A warm, salted bath is also a wonderful way to relax.) Additionally, most are not aware that vitamin K_2 (not K_1) is a potent inhibitor of muscle cramps, especially if you have night cramps. Take it before bed; it worked wonders for me.

- **Fatigue:** You may have lowered the glucose in your bloodstream by reducing the amount of carbs and protein you're consuming, but you may not have improved your fat burning enough yet to make up more of the energy that glucose had been supplying. The resulting energy deficit can lead to feelings of fatigue.

  You can use black coffee or tea with added healthy butter, coconut oil, or MCT oil to help ensure that you're getting enough fat. If your fatigue lingers for a couple of weeks, consider having a blood test to determine your carnitine levels. L-carnitine is a transporter for long-chain fatty acids, ferrying them across the inner mitochondrial membrane where they are oxidized for energy. If it's not in plentiful supply, your mitochondria will still use ketones and medium-chain fats, but oxidation of longer-chain fats slows down. Carnitine can be the key that unlocks that gate. (The jury is out as to whether or not carnitine may be problematic for people with cancer, so, if in doubt, leave it out.)

- **Heart palpitations:** This is common and is usually associated with dehydration and electrolyte loss. The remedy can be as simple as drinking a glass of water—try that first, and move on to a cup of salted broth if they don't subside. Also consider increasing magnesium and/or potassium supplementation, both of which frequently help, but check with your physician first. And if the problem persists, be certain to have it evaluated by your physician.

- **Constipation:** This is a common complaint for people in general and it can be an even bigger issue for people with cancer because prescription pain relievers, chemo, and changes in how you digest your food can all contribute to the problem. The best way to ward off constipation is to make sure you are eating plenty of fiber and staying well hydrated. You can sprinkle freshly ground flax seeds over anything you eat, and have big salads with nuts and seeds and plenty of extra virgin olive oil.

You can also soak flax seeds overnight and use them in your smoothie. Organic psyllium is another useful fiber supplement.

MCT oil is also renowned for its ability to get your bowels moving; refer back to Chapter 5 for guidance on how to introduce it slowly. If you get GI upset, go back down to a level that's comfortable and stay there. Probiotics will also help relieve constipation. It's best to get them from traditionally fermented foods, such as sauerkraut and kimchi, but a high-quality supplement can be helpful if it's challenging for you to eat fermented foods every day.

NUTRIENT-DENSE SMOOTHIE RECIPE

Makes 1 smoothie

I love using smoothies to take in a lot of nutrients in one tasty swoop. Below are the ingredients I use to make my twice-daily smoothie, which is low carb, high fat, and moderate protein. I typically include everything on this list, although it does fluctuate depending on what I have available. Don't be intimidated by the long list of ingredients. Try to incorporate everything in the foundation, and add optional add-ins as you see fit.

Foundation:

  1 teaspoon to 1 tablespoon MCT oil (depending on tolerance)
  ½ to 1 avocado (depending on preference)
  1 scoop organic greens powder
  1 tablespoon organic whole-husk psyllium
  1 to 3 ounces frozen organic fruit
  1 to 3 droppers full of stevia (to taste)
  2 tablespoons raw organic cocoa butter
  1 tablespoon organic chia seeds
  1 tablespoon flax seeds (soaked overnight)

Optional add-ins:

1 tablespoon black cumin or black sesame seeds (soaked overnight)
1 teaspoon hawthorn berries
½ teaspoon pau d'arco powder
½ teaspoon ground organic egg shells
1 teaspoon food-grade diatomaceous earth
1 teaspoon trumpet mushroom powder

Directions:

Combine everything in a blender—I use a one-quart NutriBullet. Fill with water nearly to the top. Blend for approximately two minutes. Enjoy!

MANAGING YOUR EMOTIONS DURING TRANSITION

As is true with any significant change, if you are feeling hopeful and confident, you will be better equipped to make a smooth transition to a fat-burning diet. Taking charge of your health in this way can be quite a dramatic shift from how you've dealt with health issues in the past: by simply responding to orders from your doctor. You may feel unqualified to take on this responsibility. Or, you may feel reluctant to give up bread, cookies, chips, or even foods that you once thought were healthy. Or, you may be facing a frightening medical diagnosis that has left you feeling overwhelmed or even depressed.

If you are considering this eating plan, or even reading this book, because someone who cares about you is pushing you to try it, take my advice—wait. If you make these changes simply to please someone else, you are less likely to truly commit to the eating plan. Without commitment, you are more likely to quit at the first real challenge and blame the diet, when in actuality you simply weren't ready to embrace these changes. If that's the case, let the ideas that I'm presenting in this book continue to percolate in your mind. I hope that someday in the near future you'll feel more ready to embark on this adventure.

Another peril in starting MMT while in a state of emotional turmoil is that you are more likely to turn to food for comfort or you will be easily discouraged by any little bump in the road—one high glucose reading may leave you with doubts that undermine your confidence and commitment.

> **Transition Tip:** It's normal to have some cravings when you first start MMT. These are typically easily to deal with if you are prepared with some high-fat snacks (see page 144 for ideas). If you are craving *comfort* food, however, no number of fat bombs will satisfy you. Then you need to ask yourself the question, *What else can I do that will make me feel loved and cared for?* Turning back to high-carb foods at this juncture will only prolong or derail your transition, and ultimately that's not a very loving thing to do to yourself.

Spend some time thinking about why you are making these changes. Think beyond weight loss and include improvements you want to see in your health. Write these down so you can refer back to them in moments when you're tempted to revert to old eating habits. Be specific so you can honestly assess the progress you've made.

Another powerful strategy is to visualize yourself healthy the way you want to be and attach as many positive emotions to that image as you can. Write this down and regularly reflect and meditate on this state. It is especially important to seek to experience as many of the positive emotions connected to achieving this goal as possible; this will radically increase your likelihood of attaining it.

I am also a strong advocate of the Emotional Freedom Technique (EFT) as a powerful tool to mediate emotional stressors. EFT is a DIY, needleless form of acupuncture that entails tapping on specific points on your face, arms, and hands while repeating positive affirmations. I've written about it extensively at eft.mercola.com. If you run into emotional roadblocks along your MMT journey, I highly recommend exploring EFT. You can do it on your own, or find a certified practitioner; the information I've compiled on my website will provide you with resources and help you decide on the approach that suits you best.

Exercise—but Keep It Moderate

As your body adjusts to burning fat instead of glucose as your primary fuel, it's best if you keep to moderate levels of activity. Strenuous exercise at this time can interfere with your ability to keep glucose low by breaking down muscle tissue, which is then recycled into glucose by the liver.

One way to determine if your workout was too strenuous is to measure your blood glucose before and after your exercise session. If it's higher than 10 to 20 mg/dL after your workout, you know that you've triggered the liver to manufacture more glucose. If this happens, go for a 30-minute walk (or swim or take a gentle bike ride) to allow your muscles to take up that glucose. This is preferable to leaving it in your bloodstream, where it can cause an uptick in insulin.

Walking is a fantastic form of exercise for nearly everyone. In addition to regulating your blood sugar, it reduces cytokines, signaling molecules often associated with inflammation. Walking improves mood and self-esteem, and just as importantly, the more time you spend walking, the less time you spend sitting—which is a risk factor for nearly every major chronic disease. You don't need much to reap the benefits. Multiple studies show that just a few hours of walking a week lowers the risk of breast cancer.

Most days, I walk barefoot on the beach for one to three hours and use the time to clear my thoughts, make phone calls, and go through the stack of books and journal articles stored on my Kindle—all this while deriving the health benefits of sun exposure (wearing shorts and no shirt) and grounding. By being in direct connection with the earth, you establish an electrical connection that provides positive ions stored in the ground, which can then neutralize free radicals in the body (for more information on this, please see my previous book, *Effortless Healing*). I don't consider this walk to be exercise—rather, I view it as pleasurable movement with the added benefit of reducing the risk of obesity, stroke, coronary heart disease, breast and colon cancer, type 2 diabetes, and osteoporosis while also improving mental health, blood pressure, and blood lipid profiles.[1]

I am also a strong proponent of high-intensity interval training, so I understand if you are reading this section and thinking, *No way am I only taking walks for exercise.* Remember: keeping workouts light is only temporary. Once you are through the transition process, it is likely that you will be able to return to your high-intensity workouts.

For some of Miriam's clients, maintaining high-intensity exercise despite their disease and new eating pattern is a quality-of-life issue: the thought of backing off, even if it is temporary, is enough to keep them from fully committing to needed changes. She counsels them that there are still many metabolic advantages to adopting a high-fat diet, but they need to understand that their intensive workouts can slow or even derail their progress unless it is very carefully managed and monitored. (Ketone supplementation and Peak Fasting are particularly valuable to athletes.) It is ultimately your decision to make—but you want to make it with your eyes open. The book *The Art and Science of Low-Carb Performance* is an extremely valuable guide if both a high-fat diet and high-intensity exercise are important to you.

KNOW THE CHALLENGES

After working with hundreds of clients, Miriam is acutely aware of the most common challenges people face when adopting a fat-burning eating plan. Be proactive and stand ready to face them head on and you will lessen the likelihood that any of these common issues will derail your efforts or cause your commitment to waver.

- **Variety.** Relying on a small number of foods—the same big salad at lunch, or having nuts for a snack every single day—can get old over time. It can also prompt you to seek out foods that are not part of your fat-burning eating plan. If food boredom is an issue for you, you will have to challenge yourself to try out new recipes; there are literally thousands of them at your fingertips via a simple Internet search (also, see the sidebar on page 162 for several websites with many high-fat-friendly recipes). Simply put "low carb" or "ketogenic" into a search engine along with the name of your favorite meal and you are likely to find several recipe options. Just five years ago, you couldn't find MMT-friendly recipes this easily, but the rise in popularity of this style of eating and people's willingness to share their favorites has made discovering new fat-burning snacks and meals incredibly easy. But you need to be careful and analyze the net carbs and protein, as many of these recipes will need to be modified.

- **Subtle—or not-so-subtle—social pressures.** When you are out to dinner with friends or at a party, it can be daunting or uncomfortable to explain why you're not eating the pasta, or the rice, or even the quinoa. Perhaps you're getting raised eyebrows in your own home from loved ones. It will take resolve on your part not to have "just a bite" to keep the peace. If you're attending a social event, eat before you go, or bring an MMT-friendly dish with you that everyone can enjoy, such as deviled eggs, nuts coated in butter and salt and roasted at a low heat, or a macadamia nut hummus.

   Most likely, your friends and family will need to be educated about the benefits of your plan, especially if they view it as an extreme weight-loss diet; being able to serve them something delicious can go a long way here. It helps if you keep the emphasis on the foods you *can* have, not on the foods you aren't eating. If you present your plan as a *special* diet instead of a *restrictive* diet, people may be open to learning more, and may even follow suit, especially once they see the positive changes in your health.

- **Newness of the diet.** For most people, MMT is a significant change from their usual diet. You will need to find ways to incorporate more fats when you are no longer eating things like mashed potatoes or toast with jam. It may take some time to build a new habit of reaching for vegetables and fats instead of sandwiches and chips. So it is best to start off with a limited number of simple and reliable meals so you don't get overwhelmed at every meal. You can then gradually expand your repertoire as your comfort level and desire for variety increase.

- **Environment.** Hopefully you did a pantry sweep, as I discussed in Chapter 7. But setting up your kitchen so it is easy to make MMT-friendly meals and avoid temptation from old favorites is a journey, not a destination. You may still think you need to buy chips for the kids, for example, or perhaps you only had the energy to empty out one cabinet when you got started. The thrift factor can be an issue too; many people are reluctant to rid their cabinets of food that is not spoiled and is conventionally viewed as healthy. Expect, too, that as you discover more recipes, you will realize you need a few more staples. Keep in mind that a well-stocked MMT-friendly kitchen will inspire you to keep moving forward with your plan.

- **Travel.** Whether you're going to be out all day running errands or planning a longer trip, you've got to think ahead about what you will need to have with you while you're away from home. I always travel with a set of staples, such as up to a dozen avocados to add to smoothies and salads, canned sardines or anchovies for healthy protein choices, powdered MCT oil, and a mixture of nuts and seeds along with all my supplements. I put the avocados in a cardboard tube that fits in my luggage to prevent them from being crushed. I then add them to my smoothies and salad. This volume nearly fills one checked bag but it is more than worth it to me to not be dependent on the typically terrible food choices that are available when I travel.

- **Celebrations.** Here's a common scenario: It's your birthday, and your daughter made you a cake. What do you do? You want to honor her effort, but if you eat a piece, it can derail your progress for several days, even weeks, as one transgression often begets another. In this situation, it's enough to acknowledge the effort and take the lead in cutting a piece for everyone at the party, adding, "You make such beautiful cakes! Thank you so much for thinking of me." Other times, you may be able to skirt the issue entirely by offering a suggestion as to how this special person can truly please you. For example, you may say, "What I would really love right now is a cup of tea!"

  Another option: you can prepare MMT-friendly foods (again, this is where an Internet search for "grain and sugar-free cheesecake," for example, comes in very handy). But even better, *whenever possible*, think of new ways to celebrate birthdays, holidays, and anniversaries. Keep the focus on the company and the reason for the celebration, not on any particular food.

- **Things going well.** Let's say you see your glucose readings are trending lower and you've lost some weight. It's very tempting to think you've been so successful in meeting your goals that you don't need to follow the eating plan anymore, or to get so complacent that you no longer tend to details such as weighing your intake. At these times you may need to remind yourself that there's always room for improvement. So instead of dropping out, set some new and even more ambitious goals!

Deciding how long you want to continue with the MMT eating plan depends a lot on what you expect to gain. If you have cancer, you may always want to eat this way, especially if it results in an amazing and unexpected response. Otherwise, you can basically remain on the program over the long term by following the principles of feast-famine cycling, which I cover in Chapter 10.

If you're committed to the idea of MMT but are having a rough time with these or other common challenges, or any other aspect of the eating plan, I strongly recommend you seek help from a health coach or a nutritionist who is trained in supporting high-fat diets. A professional can help you trouble-shoot your issues by asking questions about what's working and what's not and then looking at your food diary and data such as your glucose readings and making some targeted suggestions. in combination with the overall support they provide, this extra bit of coaching can make all the difference between success and failure. MMT is such a powerful plan that you want to make sure you haven't given up on it too soon, especially if the problem had an easy fix.

Often, people who seek out Miriam's help do so because they are feeling overwhelmed by all the changes. But if they already understand food basics and are comfortable with preparing meals from scratch, quite often she can get them past their trouble spots and help them feel much more confident in only three or four hours. It's not a big investment, but the payoff is huge. Another plus is that most people with extensive experience here offer their services online or through phone- or web-based video consultations.

To that end, Miriam and I have worked with Certified Nutrition Specialists to provide a training and certification course for physicians and nutritionists. You can go to their site (www.NutritionSpecialists.org) to find a consultant.

Using MMT to Optimize Conventional
Breast Cancer Treatment

In July 2015, Denise was in Hawaii, on vacation with college friends, celebrating their 60th birthdays. Drying off at the beach, she noticed what felt like a bruise on her left breast. She wasn't terribly concerned—she and her friends had been snorkeling, boogie boarding, and hiking volcanoes. Surely she'd just gotten bumped and hadn't noticed.

Fast forward to August 2016, when Denise learned she had Stage IIIA lobular breast cancer. She and her husband immediately launched into intense research mode, reading up on treatment strategies, cutting-edge breakthroughs, recurrence and survival statistics: information they would need for the many complicated choices a breast cancer patient must make. After a few weeks, they began to close in on a plan that they believed would maximize Denise's odds of survival.

By September, Denise was receiving a hormone inhibitor plus a chemo pill, therapy designed to shrink the tumor and suppress the hormones that allow some breast cancer cells to thrive. She also decided to adopt a ketogenic diet in an effort to both deny cancer its primary fuel source and to lose weight. At five feet five, Denise weighed 223 pounds. Her research had shown her that *fat itself*, especially belly fat, was her primary source of cancer-promoting hormones. She'd read the scary fact that women who did not get their weight down to a healthy range had a much higher rate of recurrence and earlier death.

Denise started working with Miriam Kalamian to develop a sensible plan for managing breast cancer. In her case, that also meant limiting estrogen-heavy dairy products, so Denise adopted a reduced-calorie, light-dairy ketogenic diet.

As Denise puts it, "I love carbs, but when faced with my own mortality, I love my husband and kids more. And I need to be here to take care of my mother, who has Alzheimer's." She adapted easily to her new plan: eggs for breakfast, avocado bacon boats for lunch, five squares of Lily's dark chocolate (sweetened with stevia) for a snack, and salad, sautéed mushrooms, and pick-your-protein for dinner. She rounded that out with blackberries or almonds and coconut for dessert. At the movies she'd have a Cocommune bar, which is "very close to an Almond Joy," she reports. At restaurants she ordered salmon, broccoli, and a salad. Instead of mashed potatoes at Thanksgiving, she served mashed cauliflower with lots of butter and it was a hit with her guests.

Denise added, "I got on with my life and believe that I'm truly, actually lengthening it with my food choices. I've dropped seventy-five pounds. I feel healthy and energetic." Even while on chemo, she restarted dance and aerobic classes. Her sleep pattern improved, and as she notes, "I look pretty dang good. And my husband jokes, 'Fighting cancer seems to agree with you.'"

No stranger to dieting, Denise was pleased to discover that cravings and hunger pangs, a bane of her past efforts at weight loss, disappeared in about 10 days, and after that, sticking to the plan was fairly easy. She does caution, "If you cheat, you've got to go through those ten very hard days again. Not worth it."

With few exceptions, Denise kept to her plan through a round of radiation in April and May of 2016, adding in intermittent fasting with the aim of reducing the side effects of treatment and increasing the cancer's sensitivity to radiation. She did so by not eating for 16 hours before each treatment. She drank a lot of water to stay hydrated but kept her food intake to a 5-hour window in the afternoon.

After drug therapy, a diet upgrade, a mastectomy, and radiation, Denise is considered cancer free. But, as with all breast cancer survivors, her recurrence risk is considered high, so Denise is likely to continue with a hormone inhibitor for five to seven years. She also plans on staying on the ketogenic diet for at least that long. Her logic: "While I'm starving any cancer remnants of hormones, why would I not starve them of carbs and sugar as well? Preventative maintenance seems crucial. I do not want to have to go through this again!" Denise's efforts have succeeded on so many fronts. Why wouldn't she want to stay with a plan that's working for her?

CHAPTER 9

USING MMT OVER THE LONG TERM

By now you should be over the hump of transition and well into the fat-burning zone. Now my goal is to provide you with guidelines and benchmarks based on my many conversations with experts on how to optimally repair your mitochondrial metabolism. It's important for you to understand that this book is merely a starting point. In order to be successful over the long term, you will need to customize MMT to meet your individual needs and unique set of goals.

This is a critical step because MMT is much more than just a diet that you follow for a few weeks until you've lost some weight or stick to for a few months to reach some other goal before reverting to your former eating habits. Once you are physiologically fat adapted, this unique approach can be a lifelong way of living, especially when you integrate feast-famine cycling, which I explain in Chapter 10. The physical and mental benefits will keep motivating you to follow this healthy plan. All you need to do is stick with it.

There may be periods when it is more challenging to strictly adhere to the plan, and I will cover these situations later in this chapter. I am confident that once you experience how much better you feel when eating this way, you will likely be hooked for the long term. This chapter will cover how to make your fat-burning status a long-term part of your life.

The Definition of Being Fat Adapted

Let's take a moment to define what it means to be fully adapted to burning fat. There are two levels.

1. Physiological Adaptation

When you first reduce your net-carb and protein intake and increase your consumption of healthy fats by following my instructions in the previous chapter, your body will naturally begin to burn more fat. It will also start converting some of that fat into clean-burning ketones that can in turn fuel most of the cells in your body, including your brain. When this happens, you are "in ketosis."

It's important to remember that it takes a while for your cells to adapt to using those ketones efficiently, as some of the enzymes required to break down ketones are different from those needed for glucose. So even though you are producing ketones when you first enter ketosis, your cells are not yet adept at using them for fuel because your body is not yet producing adequate amounts of the enzymes required to metabolize them. Adaptation can also take longer if you are older or insulin resistant or have high levels of circulating insulin, which can interfere with your ability to maintain a constant state of ketosis. If this is the case, expect it to take longer (months rather than weeks) for you to fully adapt to burning fat.

Your body needs to make other adjustments as well. As glucose levels drop, your muscles, which can already use fuels from several sources, will speed up the process at which they move fat into your mitochondria where it can be oxidized for energy. Your heart, which doesn't utilize much glucose for energy under normal conditions, uses fatty acids for fuel but will add ketones to the mix just as soon as they become available.

Your brain is more selective because it's protected by a special membrane called the blood-brain barrier, which doesn't allow large molecules, including longer-chain fats, to cross into the brain. However, small ketones can readily pass through this barrier and are then shuttled into your brain tissue using special transporters. You already have some of these transporters, but you will make more as glucose levels drop and ketone levels rise. Your brain's metabolic flexibility will gradually improve until it can harness 60 to 70 percent of its fuel from fat.

Maintaining your fat-burning ability helps keep these enzyme levels high and helps your brain tissue make better use of ketones. Because this adaptation is crucial to survival, brain tissue is able to ramp up production of the enzyme much more quickly than some other tissues. How long it will take your brain to *maximize* its use of ketones for fuel is difficult to predict and highly variable, depending on your age, your metabolic health, your genetic background, and your compliance with and response to MMT.

2. The Mental and Emotional Component

Becoming adapted to burning fat as your primary fuel is about more than your physiology. It also requires a shift in your thinking and an adjustment to your new lifestyle. Early on it might be hard to resist "sneaking" carbs, especially while you're still experiencing hunger pangs or cravings for sweet or high-net-carb foods. You might also get derailed by holidays or travel plans. Over time, though, you will be better equipped to take these challenges in stride simply because you've established new eating habits and you're firmly rooted in a new way of thinking about the connection between food and health.

You'll also enjoy the benefits of eating a high-fat, low-carb, and adequate-protein diet, and experiencing these benefits will bolster your motivation to stay with the plan. In time, these changes will no longer feel overwhelming and instead will become your "new normal." This shift in attitude and sense of yourself is an important part of the adaptation process, so be sure to give yourself enough time for this to play out

ANALYZE YOUR SUBJECTIVE DATA TO SEE HOW YOU'RE DOING

Your body is continually giving you feedback that can help guide you to your own personal fat-burning sweet spot. There is no one-size-fits-all food plan that will get you there. Although I have suggested guidelines for how much protein and net carbs to eat at each meal (see sidebar on page 211 for a recap), you may learn you need to make some changes that are a better fit for your personal situation. For example, you might lower your intake of carbs, at least for now, to stay in a fat-burning zone, or end your daily fast closer to 13 hours than to 18 hours after your last meal.

Periodically assess the following areas, and use this feedback to tailor MMT to your needs and your body.

Hunger and Cravings

As you become fat adapted, your experience of hunger will change. Your appetite won't be ruled exclusively by hormones such as insulin and glucagon, so you won't crave those foods that were formerly like opiates to your receptors. And you are far less likely get a stomach-rumbling feeling of emptiness.

Although you will still have some awareness of the need to eat, the signal won't have the urgency that comes when you are still relying on glucose as your primary source of energy. Remember: you experience the need to refuel when glucose levels drop and your brain responds by sending hormonal signals that demand your attention. This lack of urgency will in no way interfere with your enjoyment of food. You will still truly enjoy that delicious meal, but the physiological drive for it in any particular moment will not control your thoughts or actions.

If you do experience those old familiar sensations of hunger or weakness on MMT, it is probably due to one of these four conditions:

1. You are going through a period when you need more fuel than you're taking in. Perhaps, for example, you are a landscaper and it is planting season. If this is the case, the solution can be as simple as adding a few high-fat snacks. Or perhaps your weakness is related to fatigue due to illness, stress, poor sleep, or overdoing some physical activity.

2. You are Peak Fasting for too long during the day or you have not integrated the feasting cycle back into your program once you have regained the ability to burn fat as your primary fuel. This results in insulin levels actually being too low to shut down your liver's production of glucose (gluconeogenesis). You will know this is the case if your glucose levels have been consistently higher than you would expect them to be, and if when you eat 10 to 20 grams of healthy net carbs your blood sugar actually drops within the hour.

3. Adaptation is proceeding at a slower rate because your metabolism may be impaired to the point that it takes several months to a year (or even longer) before your hormones, and your body's response to them, normalizes. If this is true for you, you may be tempted to give up before you experience the benefits of MMT, so it's even more important for you to seek the counsel of a coach, metabolic doctor, or certified nutritionist who has experience with nutritional ketosis. If you have been eating a diet high in carbohydrate and protein for years, the enzymes required for burning glucose

are overexpressed, while the enzymes required for fat burning are initially not present at the levels needed for efficient utilization of fatty acids and ketones. It takes time to activate the genes to produce enough of these fat-burning enzymes. If this is your situation, you will want to seriously consider water fasting, discussed in Chapters 7 and 10.

4. If you are a woman, there are a few other factors to consider. Are your symptoms associated with a specific time in your cycle, or are you experiencing the hormone disruption common in perimenopause? How is your thyroid health? You may want to work with your health care provider to address these hormonal issues.

Energy Level

As you become adapted to burning fat for fuel, your energy will level out at a higher baseline than it was when you were burning glucose, which needed to be replenished every couple of hours. As your body makes more of the enzymes and activates other processes necessary to metabolize dietary fats and stored fats, you will have an astonishingly steady supply of energy that isn't reliant on your immediate food intake. For that reason you can assume that the consistency of your energy levels is a sign that you are in a fat-burning zone.

If your energy levels are fluctuating, it could be an indication that you are bouncing in and out of fat burning. You may be inadvertently replenishing your glycogen stores, so take a good look at how many net carbs and grams of protein you're eating. You may need to reduce those further in order to achieve consistent and long-term fat burning.

If your fatigue is sustained, refer back to Chapter 8 for information on a common culprit and how to remedy it.

Mental Clarity

If you happen to notice brain fog coming back while on MMT, check your food diary. Brain fog may be related to your food choices—eating too many net carbs or an excessive amount of protein could have cued an insulin response that has kicked you out of fat burning. If you haven't been tracking, log a few days of your food intake on Cronometer.com and see if your macronutrient targets are being met.

Poor sleep is also a common cause of mental cloudiness, as are high stress and insufficient physical activity. Another factor that could be at play is a thiamine deficiency. A high-carb diet can lower brain levels of this B vitamin, which is used up when metabolizing glucose. Your brain is a glucose hog, using about 20 percent of body energy daily, and even more if you are doing strenuous mental work. Diabetics and alcoholics in particular are typically deficient in thiamine. Neurological symptoms of mild thiamine deficiency include memory impairment, fatigue, anxiety, apathy, irritability, depression, and poor sleep.

There is also a close connection between your gut and brain, so if you are experiencing brain fog, look for things that may impact the balance of your microbiome. Antibiotics can kill off beneficial bacteria, resulting in an overgrowth of disease-causing species that are destructive to both gut and brain health. Gut-disrupting medications, such as commonly prescribed proton pump inhibitors, are also responsible for upsetting this delicate balance. The chlorine in unfiltered municipal tap water can also impair your microbiome. Brain fog also might be due to a lapse in eating fermented foods or foregoing your probiotic supplements. Or it could be the result of a sensitivity or allergy to something in your environment. Histamine intolerance comes to mind. It could even be caused by a virus or post-viral syndrome.

Antibiotics and proton pump inhibitors can also interfere with the absorption of nutrients like B_1, B_6, B_{12}, folic acid, calcium, magnesium, and zinc. All of these nutrients are required for normal brain function, and deficiencies in these nutrients can affect mental clarity.

Digestion

You will likely notice a significant improvement in your digestion, with more regular bowel movements and less bloating and reflux as you continue to follow a fat-burning diet. There are multiple reasons for these phenomena. The quality of the foods you eat on MMT is much higher than that of the processed foods that make up the typical American diet. These foods contain more fiber, which acts as food for beneficial bacteria. In addition, pathogenic bacteria, such as *H. pylori* and yeast, feed on glucose, so when you dramatically lower your consumption of sugars, you increase the growth of beneficial bacteria. This in turn suppresses the growth of disease-causing bacteria by limiting their fuel source. In fact, a 2016 autism study confirms that you may notice a significant improvement in the health of your microbiome.[1]

If you notice digestive symptoms getting worse while following MMT, or are experiencing constipation, take a careful look at your food logs (or track your food intake for a few days if you haven't been keeping regular records). Check in with your coach or health care provider for help with troubleshooting (and refer back to Chapter 8) to see if there are other explanations for what might be going on.

Chronic Conditions

The symptoms of many chronic conditions may ease up or disappear entirely as a result of the changes you make with MMT—refer to Appendix A for more specific information. This is because MMT improves mitochondrial metabolism and reduces systemic inflammation, both of which are often at the root of many chronic diseases. Be sure to work with your health care provider, as you may need to reduce or eliminate medications as your health improves. Remember: food is medicine.

Muscle Mass

Burning fat for fuel and providing your body with all its essential nutrients help you maintain your muscle mass even as you lose weight. An ideal situation is when all the weight you lose is fat rather than lean body mass. However, if you notice that you can't seem to build new muscle even with regular workouts, or that you're losing muscle tone despite eating what you perceive to be the right balance of macronutrients, it may be a sign that you need to increase your protein intake by 25 percent or even more on the days when you are doing strength training.

ALSO CONSIDER THE OBJECTIVE DATA

Balance the information you've gathered on how you're feeling with these quantifiable measurements:

Blood Glucose Levels

Over time, you should see your fasting blood glucose levels trend downward, which is a great sign because it suggests that you're giving your body a chance to regain its insulin sensitivity while also reducing systemic inflammation—two fundamental building blocks of good health.

If your glucose levels aren't trending downward, or you experience substantial, unexplained inconsistencies from day to day, refer back to page 179 for a list of possible reasons and remedies.

Ketones

Remember that unless you are addressing an ongoing chronic disease, you really only need to monitor your ketone levels in the first few weeks or months of your program, and then occasionally as a check on whether your plan is still working for you. Ideally, blood levels of ketones will range between 0.5 and 3.0 mmol/L.

I suggest checking your ketone levels either with a home blood ketone test or a breath meter tester like the Ketonix. I use a Ketonix to check my ketones every morning to confirm I am still in ketosis, even after feasting days of 150 grams of net carbs. Remember that being in ketosis is a signal that your body is burning fat for fuel.

As I covered in Chapter 2, ketones themselves aren't the main reason why a high-fat diet has such a remarkable impact on metabolic health. It's the nutrients you consume in combination with the times when you consume them that trigger multiple beneficial chain reactions. Ketones are merely a by-product of this process; using them as your primary gauge of success is a little like grading a student based on how many used-up pens and pencils you find in the trash. It's about the inputs, not just the outputs— and all that happens in between.

Ketones are not the primary driver of health-promoting changes. You can make lots of ketones just from ingesting MCT oil, but unless you make changes to the rest of your diet, you will only experience a tiny fraction of benefits that a high-fat, low-carbohydrate, adequate-protein diet provides.

Your Weight—If Weight Loss Is a Goal

After the initial quick water weight loss that comes when you reduce insulin and deplete your glycogen stores (and release the water that is stored with glycogen), you will see your weight trend downward until you reach your ideal weight. That's because a calorie isn't a calorie when you are burning fat in the same way it is when you are burning glucose.

When you primarily burn glucose, your body stays mostly in fat-storage mode. But when you're burning fat for your primary fuel, your body will convert some of those fats to ketones and excrete those that aren't used through the urine. Insulin is the storage hormone and in MMT this mechanism isn't triggered as often, so it becomes easier to maintain and even lose weight.

Also, as you burn more fat rather than store it, hunger pangs ease and you lose your cravings for processed and sugary foods, making fat loss easier to achieve. If you are already at a low body weight, you'll need to make sure that you get plenty of calories from fat, enough to stabilize where you are, or even to gain a few pounds if that's what you need.

In addition to tracking your total body weight over time, I suggest weighing yourself every few days at the same time of day, after your bowel movement in the morning and before you eat your first meal or drink any fluids. You'll also want to update your estimate of body fat percentage; seeing it go down over time will help keep you motivated. (Refer to page 120 for ways to do this.)

This will also help you keep tabs on your lean body mass, which you want to keep stable or even slightly increase over time. If you embark on a muscle-building workout regimen, expect your lean body mass to increase; when that happens you will need to increase your protein intake slightly. If you are eating a well-designed high-fat diet but your lean body mass *declines* over time, I suggest working with a health coach who is well versed in ketosis on fine-tuning your program or diet while keeping to the guideline of 1 gram of protein per kilogram of lean body mass. (I suggest working with a coach well versed in high-fat, low-carb, and adequate-protein diets, because most traditional fitness trainers overprescribe protein.)

Cronometer Records

Over time, recording what you eat in a typical day becomes one of the most powerful tools you have in keeping to your MMT plan. Recording your biometrics is another essential part of your recording.

Some people embrace the most intensive approach by weighing and tracking every morsel of food they put in their mouth by using Cronometer.com/mercola, while others are more reluctant to take the time to do so. To ensure that you stay on track with your diet, aim to record at least one typical day of eating and exercise each week.

Using Cronometer will help you comply with the diet because the thought of recording every handful of chips or piece of birthday cake can influence whether you choose to eat it. It's also a continual learning tool that can help you identify which meals and foods provide the biggest bang for your nutritional buck. Using Cronometer on a regular basis will keep you from veering off track.

Cronometer can also help you assess your typical nutrient intake so you can easily see if there are any gaps you need to shore up with different choices or maybe even supplements.

You may find that over time, you need to restrict the amount of nonfiber carbs you are eating in order to improve on your fasting blood glucose, or that you can add more nonfiber carbs according to a feast-famine schedule, which I cover in Chapter 10, while still maintaining fat burning.

It's also helpful to use Cronometer to track a few micronutrient ratios. In particular you'll want to keep your eye on these ratios:

- **Omega-6 to Omega-3:** An ideal ratio lies somewhere between 5:1 and 1:1, but this can be very hard to achieve. Certainly aim to keep this ratio at a maximum of 5:1, and keep experimenting with your diet and your omega-3 supplementation until you can settle into a more desirable 3:1 or 2:1 omega-6-to-omega-3 ratio. Ideally, it would be best to test your levels with an omega-3 index or comprehensive fatty acid profile from Quest or Lab Corp.

  Omega-3 fatty acids are one of the best ways to counter inflammation because they provide your body with chemicals called resolvins. These remarkable substances turn off inflammation in your body when it is no longer needed to fight infections.

  One caveat to keep in mind is that many have over-consumed fish oil and driven up their levels of eicosapentaenoic acid (EPA), a particular type of omega-3 fatty acid. When you take large amounts of EPA from supplements like fish oil, the level of arachidonic acid (AA) in relation to EPA can be driven down. When AA is low it can contribute to unstable cell membranes and bleeding. Life is a balance, and you need some AA for cellular structure, support, and signaling. For this reason, it's best to get your DHA from seafood or whole seafood supplements like krill oil, not isolated extracted supplements like fish oils. Healthy seafood is a superior option to krill oil, but the oil is helpful when healthy seafood is not available. Krill oil is also far better absorbed because, unlike fish oil, it is in emulsified phospholipid form.

- **Potassium to Sodium:** While sodium is often vilified as a contributor to high blood pressure and heart disease, it's not that sodium in and of itself is bad. It's that it is typically consumed in far higher amounts than its natural counterbalance—potassium.

  Potassium helps offset the hypertensive effects of sodium and helps your body maintain proper pH levels. In an article published in the *New England Journal of Medicine* in 1985, the authors evaluated the dietary intake of our Paleolithic ancestors to find they naturally consumed about 11,000 mg of potassium and 700 mg of sodium a day.[2] This equates to nearly 16 times more potassium than sodium. Today that ratio is reversed: the daily potassium intake averages 2,500 mg and sodium 3,400 mg.

  To bring your potassium intake up higher than sodium, prioritize the MMT-friendly foods that are high in potassium, including spinach, broccoli, Brussels sprouts, avocados, asparagus, nuts, and seeds. The ideal ratio of potassium to sodium you're looking for is twice as much potassium as sodium. For most people this is about 5 grams of potassium a day. Please note that the potassium needs to come from sources such as vegetables, not potassium salts, to provide health benefits.

- **Calcium to Magnesium:** Magnesium is the fourth most abundant mineral in your body. More than 3,750 magnesium-binding sites have been detected on human proteins,[3] and it's required for more than 300 different enzymes in your body—enzymes that allow you to manufacture protein, DNA, RNA, and mitochondrial energy. Magnesium is critical for the optimization of your mitochondria.

  Magnesium also functions as a counterbalance to calcium—and too much calcium with too little magnesium can lead to heart attacks, strokes, and sudden death. Your target magnesium to calcium ratio is 1:1.

  Luckily, magnesium is found in good amounts in many of the same foods that contain potassium, including leafy greens, nuts, seeds, broccoli, and Brussels sprouts, as well as cacao powder (good news if you're a fan of chocolate fat bombs). The recommended dietary allowance for magnesium[4] ranges from 310 to 420 mg per day, depending on your age and sex. However, I and many researchers believe we may need anywhere from 600 to 900 mg/day for optimal health.

- **Fiber to Calories:** As I covered in Chapter 5, I recommend that you consume at least 35 to 50 grams of fiber, ideally from fresh, locally grown organic vegetables, nuts, and seeds. If you fall short of the recommended amount, supplementing with organic psyllium husk can help you reach this target.

If you aren't meeting your targets for these nutrients, troubleshoot them sooner rather than later. Work with someone who can be objective, such as a coach who can review your food intake logs and blood test results and help pinpoint where you can make some improvements.

Cholesterol Levels

Perhaps 25 to 30 percent of people who adopt a high-fat diet will experience an initial rise in triglyceride and cholesterol levels. In others, the levels stay the same or even drop. There are a few factors to consider in deciding for yourself whether this should be a cause for concern:

- The link between cholesterol and cardiovascular disease isn't as solid as conventional medicine holds. Research published in 1996 found that 50 percent of heart attack victims and 80 percent of patients with coronary artery disease have normal cholesterol levels.

- LDL-C, the most common test to assess serum levels of LDL particles, is actually just an estimate of the number of particles, and like most estimates is subject to error.

- Even when LDL cholesterol rises, long-term observations of children on the diet for epilepsy note that it often but not always returns to near pre-diet levels after 6 to 12 months. This return to baseline levels appears true for adults as well.

- LDL cholesterol is usually viewed as "bad." As I noted in Chapter 1, it is made up of two types of particles: one type (Pattern B) that is small and dense, and may contribute to atherosclerosis, and another type (Pattern A) that is large and light and less likely to have a harmful effect on your arteries. So even if LDL does rise, unless the test is one of the newer and more sophisticated lipid panels that calculate numbers of both types of particles, this information by itself tells you very little.

- Triglycerides appear to be a better indicator of the true risk of cardiovascular disease. Most people experience a dramatic *drop* in triglyceride levels after starting a high-fat diet, mostly because excessive carbohydrates are the primary cause of high levels. If levels do rise, this is usually temporary while your body makes the transition to burning fat. A reduction in carbohydrate intake is what triggers the release of triglycerides stored in fat, which can then be burned for fuel. That's why fasting before your test is so important; the triglycerides released the day before will be used as fuel during your overnight fast.

- If there is a rise in triglycerides, it is likely that it is temporary, and in most people, it will return to pre-diet levels in one to two years, according to *The Ketogenic and Modified Atkins Diets* by Kossoff et al.—an evidence-based book written by ketogenic diet specialists at Johns Hopkins Hospital.

- As I covered in Chapter 8, you may be low in carnitine, which shuttles long-chain fatty acids across mitochondrial membranes. Because a high-fat diet requires more carnitine than a traditional diet, your levels may drop. This can be identified with a blood test to measure your free carnitine levels. If your levels are indeed low *and* you are experiencing symptoms such as fatigue or low levels of ketones, you may choose to supplement with carnitine, but work with your doctor or other health care provider before you make that decision, as evidence is mixed on whether carnitine supplementation may contribute to cancer progression. (There is more info on supplementing with carnitine in Chapter 11.)

- Certain medications can affect your blood lipid levels, and you should take this into consideration when deciding whether or not the diet is working for you. Lack of sleep, illness, and high levels of stress can impact your numbers.

- If you are facing a dire diagnosis, such as an aggressive cancer, you have to decide what's more important— starving the disease that is threatening your life, or keeping your blood lipid levels within a range that has been determined to be normal even though those norms are based on an unhealthy population.

If you do experience a rise in blood lipid levels or if you are confused or discouraged by a change in your lipid levels, please reach out to a health coach or other health care provider who specializes in high-fat, low-carb diets so you can get some objective insight into your situation before you give up on the plan.

Basic Guidelines for Optimum Fat Burning over the Long Term

These guidelines are a starting point and can vary widely based on your current health, health goals, and life circumstances. You will have to discover the benchmarks that work best for you.

Fasting blood glucose: Below 80

Ketones: Above .5 mmol/L, or consistently some shade of pink if you're using urine test strips. If you are using the Ketonix breath instrument, if you see a flashing red light you know you are in ketosis; the more flashes, the deeper the level of ketosis.

Formula for determining protein needs: 1 gram per kilogram of lean body mass unless you are pregnant, breast-feeding, a competitive athlete, or elderly, as individuals in these groups may require additional protein.

Max amount of protein from both animal and plant sources in any one meal: 12 to 15 grams for most women (unless pregnant or nursing—then you may need more), 15 to 20 grams for most men.

MMT macronutrient ratios (may vary): 50 to 85 percent fat[*]; 4 to 32 percent carbs; 8 to 12 percent protein[†].

Peak Fasting duration: 13 to 18 hours.

---

[*]   Once you are able to easily generate ketones, you can drop your percentage of fat calories to 50 percent and replace them with more net carbs from whole foods—not grains—so long as you retain fat-burning ability, measured by your ability to keep your ketone levels above about .5 mmol/L.

[†]   The only time you'd want to consider increasing your protein levels above this suggested range is if you are strength training or otherwise aiming to increase muscle mass.

CHAPTER 10

THE POWER OF FASTING TO OPTIMIZE MITOCHONDRIAL HEALTH

In previous sections of this book I have thoroughly covered how foods can optimally support your mitochondria and dramatically improve your health. But eating even the best health-promoting foods is only half the equation when it comes to taking care of your health in general and your mitochondria in particular.

By focusing too much on what foods to eat, we forget that eating has a natural and powerful counterbalance, which is *not* eating.

Everything in nature has two sides: darkness and light, activity and rest, hot and cold. Fasting is the flip side of eating—as Dr. Jason Fung, the co-author of *The Complete Guide to Fasting* and

The Obesity Code calls it—and fasting plays a vitally important role in allowing your body to function at its best.

Why? Because your body simply isn't designed to run optimally when it is continuously fed.

If regularly going without food were detrimental to human health, we certainly wouldn't have survived, let alone flourished as a species. Humans have evolved to not only withstand extended periods where food isn't available, but to thrive *because* they didn't have continuous access to food as many of us now do in the 21st century.

Yet this isn't what we've been led to believe. The media, conventional medicine, and the food industry have drilled it into us that we need to eat all day long. These statements have been repeated so often that we've come to believe that they're true: breakfast is the most important meal of the day; you need to eat three square meals plus snacks to keep your metabolism high; eating a snack before bedtime helps you sleep.

But we haven't always lived with food available 24/7. As Fung describes fasting in *The Complete Guide to Fasting*, "Fasting is the oldest dietary intervention in the world. It is not just the latest and greatest, but the tried and true."

Water or Fat Fasting

At the present time more than two out of three adults in our population are overweight or obese,[1] and that number is steadily climbing. This tragedy is also ravaging the health of our children. It makes perfect sense for those who are overweight to consider an extended fast. Periods of fasting can range from a few days to a few weeks. Not only will this simplify the program for most people, but it will also rapidly accelerate the transition to fat burning and immediately begin to improve metabolic pathways that address the fundamental causes of many health challenges. Hunger pangs and cravings can be a challenge on days two and three, but after that the cravings tend to dramatically decrease.

Being adapted to burning fat before even starting a well-designed nutritional ketosis plan may even improve your implementation because by the time you start, you'll have passed the point where hunger and cravings can undermine your efforts. An interesting alternative that may make the process even easier is to consume healthy fats while keeping carbs and protein under 5 grams of each per day. Since carbs and protein are really the only macronutrients that activate mTOR, insulin, leptin, and IGF-1, by virtually eliminating them you can obtain most of the benefits of water fasting yet not experience the typical loss of energy. Examples of fats you can use are healthy pastured butter, coconut oil, and MCT oil in a hot beverage of tea or coffee. You can add naturally processed stevia to make the drink more palatable, although most people following this type of diet no longer crave sweet. Most find this a much easier alternative to water fasting.

Whatever type of fast you choose, water or fat, once you have completed it you will need to transition to foods with low net carbs, low protein, and high-quality fats. This transition is typically much easier in those who have achieved fat burning and nutritional ketosis using these fasts.

If you are interested in implementing this approach or even just intrigued enough to learn more, I strongly encourage you to obtain a copy of *The Complete Guide to Fasting*. It is a comprehensive guide that will serve as a valuable resource for anyone considering this approach.

Fasting is a ritual that is an integral part of nearly every major religious tradition—Jesus, Buddha, and Muhammad all observed fasts that played a large role in their spiritual transformations. Hippocrates was the father of medicine, and he recommended that overweight people eat only once a day. Benjamin Franklin wrote, "The best of all medicines is resting and fasting." And even Mark Twain was a fasting proponent, having written, "A little starvation can really do more for the average sick man than can the best medicines and the best doctors."

It's only recently that we've lost touch with the power of fasting to heal, in large part because it was only within the last century that humans learned to manipulate the food supply through agriculture and long-distance transportation to the point that food became available in abundance 24/7 and all year long. Although there clearly are exceptions, it appears a large part of humanity regularly went through some periods of starvation or famine.

Research reveals that a vast majority of Americans eat *all day long*[2]—with as many as 15.5 separate eating events in a typical day. Most also consume a majority of their daily calories late in the evening, which is exactly when your body requires the *least* amount of energy as calories from food. That's why I recommend you avoid eating for at least three hours before bedtime—and that includes *everyone*, no matter what kind of diet you follow or don't follow. This continuous access to food prevents your body from undergoing the repair and rejuvenation processes that occur during fasting.

THE SURPRISING BENEFITS OF FASTING

Fasting, much like exercise, is a biological stressor that initiates metabolic processes that promote overall health. By reintroducing periods of time without food into your daily life and mimicking the eating habits of your ancestors who did not have access to food around the clock, you can restore your body to a more natural state that allows a whole host of biochemical benefits to occur.

Physiologically, the benefits of fasting include:

- **Blood sugar stabilizes.** Because you aren't taking in calories, blood glucose levels fall to normal fasting levels, well below 100. They also stabilize, as the liver begins producing glucose via the process of gluconeogenesis, at least in nondiabetics.

- **Insulin levels lower and insulin resistance is improved.** Because blood glucose levels fall, your body doesn't need to release as much insulin to shuttle glucose out of the bloodstream and into the cells, so insulin levels also fall, allowing your body to heal from insulin resistance.

- **The gut and the immune system get a change to rest.** Fasting allows the digestive tract to rest and regenerate the mucosal lining. Also, the immune system is not under the continual stress of addressing a constant stream of food antigens, which allows the immune system to participate in regeneration of the body's organs. In addition, short fasts will trigger the activation of stem cells to produce new white blood cells, which boosts immunity.

- **Ketones are produced.** Since ketones provide an alternative source of energy, they also preserve muscle mass. And of course, they provide a needed alternative to glucose for the brain and central nervous system.

- **Metabolic rate increases.** Your levels of adrenaline rise to provide energy in the absence of food, meaning your overall metabolic rate is actually increased (as opposed to the myth of fasting that says it suppresses metabolism and puts your body into "starvation mode").

- **Damaged cells are cleared out.** Fasting triggers autophagy, a natural cleansing routine your body uses to clean out cellular debris, including toxins, while also recycling damaged cell components. Autophagy, which, as you learned in Chapter 2, translates as "self-eating," contributes to many important functions by helping your stem cells retain the ability to maintain and repair your tissues,[3] dampening inflammation, slowing down the aging process, slowing the growth of cancer, and optimizing biological function.

- **Hunger lessens.** Contrary to popular belief, once you adjust to fasting, your subjective feelings of hunger are reduced. Why? In large part because fasting lowers levels of insulin and leptin, and improves both insulin and leptin receptor sensitivity. Both of these important metabolic improvements help mobilize the oxidation of fat stores and other major hormonal drivers of obesity and chronic disease.

- **Excess body fat is shed.** In my 30 years of clinical practice, I saw firsthand that intermittent fasting was one of the most effective—and easiest—ways to rid yourself of excess body fat without losing lean body mass. When you go for an extended period without eating, you consume fewer overall calories, meaning that body composition is naturally regulated to optimal proportions. You may eat a large meal once you break your fast, but studies show that first meal contains only 20 percent more calories than an average meal: not enough to negate the calories that you *didn't* eat during your fast.[4]

  A small pilot study evaluated the efficacy of intermittent fasting in reducing weight in humans. In this study, *the only* dietary change made was restricting eating to a 10- to 12-hour window each day. For the remaining 12 to 14 hours, participants fasted. After four months, those who had fasted daily had lost an average of more than seven pounds. And, while they were not specifically instructed to cut calories, they ended up reducing their daily calories by an average of 20 percent anyway.[5]

- **Reduces levels of hormones thought to promote cancer.** Taking regular breaks from food intake not only reduces levels of insulin and leptin, but also insulin-like growth factor 1 (IGF-1), a potent hormone that acts on your pituitary gland to induce powerful metabolic and endocrine effects, including cell growth and replication.

  Elevated IGF-1 levels are associated with many cancers, including breast and prostate cancers. Cancer cells have more receptors for this hormone than normal cells, and reducing levels of IGF-1 is associated with reduced cell proliferation in many cancers. Fasting also reduces levels of pro-inflammatory cytokines, small proteins that also have a role in promoting cancer.

- **The rate of aging slows.** In addition to boosting levels of human growth hormone, fasting decreases the accumulation of free radicals in your cells, thereby preventing the oxidative damage to cellular proteins, lipids, and DNA. This damage is strongly associated with aging and most chronic diseases.

    Fasting also inhibits the mammalian target of rapamycin (mTOR) pathway, which you may recall from Chapter 3 is an ancient cellular signaling pathway that orchestrates insulin, leptin, and IGF-1 and is ultimately responsible for either growth or repair, depending on whether it is stimulated or inhibited. Inhibiting mTOR is precisely your goal if your intention is to up-regulate maintenance and repair, boost longevity, and reduce your risk for cancer. This means it is a good idea for nearly everyone except bodybuilders or competitive athletes.

- **Boosts fat burning.** When you eat all day long, you never need to call on your stores of glycogen (stored glucose). Yet when you go at least 18 hours without food if you aren't already burning fat as your primary fuel, or 13 hours if you are, your liver's glycogen stores become radically depleted. At that point, your body is forced to turn to your stored fat for energy—and here begins the fat-burning state you want to remain in on the MMT eating plan.

- **Protects brain function.** Fasting can also have a very beneficial impact on your brain function, and may even hold the key to preventing Alzheimer's disease and other chronic brain disorders. Mark Mattson, Ph.D., has conducted animal studies showing that when mice that are genetically engineered to develop

Alzheimer's disease are put on an alternate-day fasting diet, they don't develop the disease until around the age of 2 years, which in human terms is equivalent to being 90.[6]

Without any intervention, the mice develop dementia in half that time or around 1 year, equivalent to the age of 40 or 50 in humans. And when Mattson put them on a junk food diet, they developed Alzheimer's disease at around 9 months!

Mattson's research suggests that alternate-day fasting can boost a protein known as brain-derived neurotrophic factor (BDNF) by anywhere from 50 to 400 percent, depending on the brain region. BDNF activates brain stem cells to convert into new neurons. It also triggers other chemicals that promote neural health and has been shown to protect brain cells from adverse changes associated with Alzheimer's disease and Parkinson's disease.[7]

A Quick Overview of What Happens in Your Body in a Fed versus a Fasted State

What Happens in the Body When You Eat	What Happens in the Body When You Fast
Energy (aka fat) is stored	Energy (aka fat) is burned
Insulin rises	Insulin falls
Human growth hormone is suppressed	Human growth hormone is released
Free radical production is increased	Free radical production goes down

The only other strategy that has so many research-backed benefits for longevity is long-term calorie restriction, which requires a significant long-term reduction in the amount of food you eat so that you are essentially living on the brink of starvation. As you probably know, compliance with calorie-restricted diets is abysmal. The good news is that there are many ways to fast, and there is likely a form of fasting out there that you will be able to tolerate and incorporate into your life without undue hardship. I'll cover these options in just a moment. It's important for you to remember that fasting can provide nearly identical benefits without the pain, suffering, and compliance challenges of calorie restriction.

Instead of regulating *how much* food you eat, as with long-term calorie restriction, you only need to modify *when* you eat—and of course wisely choose the foods you do eat. Simply cycling between periods of eating and fasting on a daily, weekly, or monthly schedule has been shown to provide many of the same benefits as long-term calorie restriction. Choosing when to eat and when to fast in this way is known as "intermittent fasting." As my colleague and fasting advocate Dr. Dan Pompa notes, "Don't eat less—eat less often."

A Tour of the Different Types of Intermittent Fasting

Intermittent fasting is rapidly gaining in popularity for the simple reason that it works. It does so whether you're trying to lose excess body fat or improve biomarkers for optimal health. As a general rule, intermittent fasting involves cutting calories, in whole or in part, either a couple of days a month or a week, every other day, or even daily, as in the case of the Peak Fasting regimen, the form of scheduled eating I prefer to use myself.

There are many ways to fast, from consuming nothing but water for two to three days each month to eating a normal amount of calories every day but during a restricted window of time so you still get a good long stretch without food intake during each 24-hour period.

The "right" fast for you is the one you will actually comply with. Here's a tour through the different options:

2- to 3-Day Water Fast

For most healthy people I am not an advocate of going without food for any period longer than about 18 hours. However, if you are overweight and have serious health challenges, a medically supervised water fast may be appropriate.

A water fast is just what it sounds like. You consume nothing but water and some minerals for a finite period of time. This type of fast can give you a shorter transition into fat burning because you will rapidly burn through your glycogen stores and push your body to start using fat for energy.

This may be appropriate for you if you have just received a very serious diagnosis, such as brain cancer. But if you are limited by any of the following conditions, consult with your health care team before embarking on this type of fast:

- Already underweight
- Nutritionally compromised
- Taking diuretics or blood pressure medications
- Have low blood pressure
- Have diabetes, thyroid disease, chronically low sodium levels, or cardiovascular disease

5-Day Fast

This is the approach proposed by Dr. Michael Mosley, author of *The Fast Diet*. He recommends that you spend five consecutive days of each month on a modified fast. You do not abstain from food entirely during these days. On the first day, you eat about 1,000 to 1,100 calories, followed by 725 calories on the remaining four days. As with all fasting options, the foods you do eat should be low in net carbohydrates and protein, and high in healthy fats.

In one 2015 experiment,[8] people who fasted five consecutive days once a month for three consecutive months saw improvements in biomarkers for cell regeneration. Risk factors for diabetes, cancer, cardiovascular disease, and aging also declined.

Beware that it can be quite challenging to go for a full five days with very little food, especially if you've never fasted before, so you may want to work your way up slowly to this type of a fast.

1-Day Fast

In this case you skip eating for one day of every week, consuming only water on that day. Your fast should be broken with a regular-sized meal (i.e., avoid eating a meal that is more than 20 percent larger than your typical meal when coming off your fast), and you can maintain your regular exercise program without any special diet recommendations for workout days.

Fasting for 24 hours can be tough for some people, but eating a high-fat, low-carb diet can make a 24-hour fast easier, as a higher-fat diet will tend to normalize your hunger hormones and provide improved satiety for longer periods of time. You can also fast from dinner to dinner, skipping a full 24 hours of eating while still eating each day.

Alternate-Day Fasting

This program is exactly as it sounds: one day off, one day on. On fasting days you restrict your eating to one meal of about 500 calories. On nonfasting days, you can eat normally.

When you include sleeping time, your fast can end up being as long as 32 to 36 hours. According to Krista Varady, Ph.D., author of *The Every-Other-Day Diet*, alternate-day fasting can help you lose up to two pounds of body fat per week.

Another benefit to alternate-day fasting is that your body tends to adapt to the regularity of the program, whereas the randomness of the 5:2 plan can be more difficult to adjust to.[9] In clinical trials, about 90 percent of participants were able to stick to alternate-day fasting, whereas the other 10 percent dropped out within the first two weeks.

I should note that I am not a fan of this type of fasting. I believe there are far better approaches with higher compliance rates. Alternate-day fasting may also diminish diastolic reserve in the heart, as one rodent study[10] found to occur in those animals that were kept on this type of fasting long term.

5:2 Fasts

Another fasting plan espoused by Dr. Michael Mosley in his book *The Fast Diet* is the 5:2 plan, where you cut your food down to one-fourth of your normal daily calories—about 600 calories for men and about 500 for women—on two days of your choice each week. On the other five days of the week you eat normally.

One thing to be aware of is that there is some evidence that the irregularity of the 5:2 plan may disrupt the circadian rhythm of your body. These automatic rhythms orchestrate your sleep/wake cycle and various functions of your hormonal system.

Peak Fasting—My Preferred Form of Intermittent Fasting

As a general rule I recommend a specific type of intermittent fasting that I call Peak Fasting. This is my hands-down favorite form of fasting and the one I personally use. It is by far the easiest to maintain once your body has shifted over from burning sugar to burning fat as its primary fuel, and it also appears to support steady circadian rhythms.

Peak Fasting is done every day rather than a few days per week or month. However, you can certainly cycle in off days to suit your schedule or social commitments—this flexibility is another major benefit of Peak Fasting. If circumstances allow, I recommend doing this type of fasting about five days a week. The process is quite simple.

The crux of Peak Fasting is to restrict your eating each day to a 6- to 11-hour window. As a result you will avoid eating for 13 to 18 hours of every day. The simplest way to implement Peak Fasting is to stop eating at least three hours before bed and then delay your first meal of the following day until at least 13 hours have passed since you last ate. A powerful illustration of its value is a recent study showing that women who fast for 13 or more hours after the evening meal may reduce the risk of early-stage breast cancer coming back.[11] It is important to note that you if you have trained your body to burn fat as your primary fuel, you have greater access to this type of benefit with an intermittent fast of only 13 hours. If you are still burning carbs as your primary fuel, it will take closer to 18 hours of fasting to achieve this benefit.

This may seem like an awfully long time to go without eating on a daily basis, but once you have transitioned to burning fat as your primary source of fuel, you won't experience those frequent hunger pangs. Another benefit of Peak Fasting is that you will be able to go for hours without a dip in energy because fat provides a continuous source of fuel. This is in contrast to glucose, which triggers glucose/insulin spikes, frequent hunger pangs, and energy crashes as cues to consume more high-carb foods.

Transition Tip: If it's difficult for you to go 13 or more hours without eating, try adding a teaspoon or two of coconut or MCT oil to a cup of coffee or tea. The fat will help ward off hunger without causing a rise in blood sugar. It essentially allows you to extend your fast while minimizing your hunger.

THE BENEFITS OF AVOIDING EATING HOURS BEFORE YOU GO TO BED

No matter which fasting program you choose, or even if you choose not to adopt any formal type of fasting, you'll want to stop eating at least three hours before you go to bed. I have recently become much more aware of how important this simple change is in helping to optimize your mitochondrial function and prevent cellular damage. Many factors influence why you will reap health benefits if you develop the habit of not eating within three hours of bedtime:

- When you are sleeping, your energy needs are at their lowest, and providing excess fuel at this time will result in the production of excessive amounts of damaging free radicals.

- Sleep is your body's time for detox and repair, and needing to digest a meal during sleep will impair these important processes.

- Nighttime is a common time for your body to use ketones for energy, since glycogen stores are typically depleted within 18 hours (13 hours if you are eating low carb), and eating too close to bedtime can replenish glycogen stores and prevent the body from burning fat for overnight fuel.

- Not eating for at least three hours before bed enables you to extend that period of time without eating food on a daily basis, making Peak Fasting an easy and rewarding way of life.

A review paper published in 2011[12] provides much of the experimental work supporting the advice to refrain from eating too close to bedtime. The take-home message is clear: since your body uses the least amount of calories when sleeping, you'll want to avoid eating close to bedtime because adding excess fuel at this time will generate excessive free radicals that will damage your tissues, accelerate aging, and contribute to chronic disease.

For this reason, I believe one of the best strategies for reducing mitochondrial free radical production is to limit the amount of fuel you feed your body when it requires the least amount, which is when you are sleeping. That's why I stop eating four to six hours before I go to bed, although a three-hour window is also beneficial and probably more doable for most people.

CONTRAINDICATIONS FOR FASTING

Although I believe intermittent fasting, particularly Peak Fasting, is a powerful way to improve your physiological function all the way down to the mitochondrial level, it is not for everyone. Individuals taking medications, especially diabetics, need medical supervision; otherwise there is a risk of hypoglycemia.

If you have serious adrenal challenges or chronic renal disease, are living with chronic stress (adrenal fatigue), or have cortisol dysregulation, you would likely need to resolve these issues before implementing intermittent fasting. Also, if you have a disease called porphyria, you should not fast.

If your goal is to build large muscles or engage in competitive sports such as sprinting that require glucose for anaerobic fast twitch muscle fibers, intermittent fasting is not likely to be your best strategy.

Pregnant women and nursing mothers should not practice intermittent fasting, as the baby needs a wider range of nutrients during and after birth, and there's no research supporting the safety of fasting during this important time.

Children under 18 should also not fast for extended periods. And anyone of any age with concerns about malnutrition, or who is underweight (with a body mass index, or BMI, of less than 18.5), or who has an eating disorder such as anorexia nervosa should avoid fasting.

When implementing intermittent fasting, keep your eye on any signs of hypoglycemia, or low blood sugar, which include:

- Light-headedness
- Shakiness
- Confusion
- Fainting
- Excessive sweating
- Blurred vision
- Slurred speech

- Feelings of an atypical heartbeat
- Pins and needles sensation in the fingertips

If you suspect that your blood sugar is low, make sure to eat something that will not impact your blood glucose levels, such as coconut oil in black coffee or tea.

Paradoxically, Peak Fasting is part of the solution for normalizing adrenal function, but you may require professional guidance to help you navigate that course if you struggle with this problem.

Tips for Adapting to a Regular Fasting Schedule

The toughest part of any intermittent fasting plan is getting through the initial transition, which can take anywhere from a week to two months. In some people this transition may take even longer, depending on how insulin resistant they are and other factors such as weight, blood pressure, and how consistent they are with their fasting regimen.

About 10 percent of people report headaches as a side effect when they first start fasting, but the biggest complaint is hunger. This is why it is so important to keep hydrated, especially while adding extra magnesium. It may also be helpful to remember that one reason you're craving food is because your body has not yet made the switch from burning sugar to burning fat as its primary fuel. As long as you're running on sugar, frequent hunger pangs will be the norm. Fat is far more satisfying, as it's a much slower-burning fuel.

Another factor that can trip you up during the transition period is purely psychological. If you're used to grazing in the evenings, it may take some time to break the habit. One trick to make it easier to go longer periods of time without eating is to drink more water. Oftentimes people mistake thirst for hunger.

It typically takes a few days to work up to 13 hours, but once you start activating your fat-burning system you will easily achieve this. The most effective way is to keep to your fat-burning plan by limiting your net carbs to under 40 grams per day and not exceeding more than 1 gram of protein per kilogram of lean body mass.

Once you achieve the ability to burn fat as your primary fuel, you will want to add some variety to this regimen, as I discuss in the feast-famine cycling section below.

Use Feast-Famine Cycling to Reap the Benefits of Fat Burning over the Long Haul without Feeling Deprived

As I have shown in this book, switching to burning fat as your primary fuel is a very powerful intervention that can improve the health of your mitochondria, which in turn improves your overall health. But you may be wondering, *How long should I keep to this eating plan?*

Many aspects of MMT are important parts of a lifelong commitment to better health, such as choosing high-quality fats, avoiding GMO foods, and eating local, organic produce whenever possible. You may believe that this is a way of eating that you could embrace for a lifetime, and for some that might be optimal. But my best guess is that is not the case for nearly everyone.

After implementing this plan for over six months, I learned that some of the metabolic changes it creates may not be beneficial over the course of a lifetime. This is mostly related to the hormone insulin and the way insulin works.

Most health professionals have been taught that insulin works by driving glucose into the cell. It turns out this is not the primary mechanism of insulin—it actually drives glucose *out* of the cell.

How can it be then that when you inject someone with insulin, especially someone who has never received insulin injections, their blood sugar will drop?[13]

It turns out the way insulin really works is to suppress gluconeogenesis—the process your liver uses to produce glucose. The reason this is not widely appreciated is that very few people actually have insulin levels low enough to stop the liver's production of glucose. About the only times this happens is during prolonged fasting and nutritional ketosis with low-net-carb intakes.

When your insulin levels are very low, your blood sugar will start to rise because your liver starts making glucose. What is really astonishing is that when you are in this state and you eat a small amount of carbs, your blood sugar will actually drop! This is because the liver is making more glucose than you are consuming and the carbohydrate you ate was enough to raise insulin levels, which then stopped the gluconeogenesis process.

I have worn a continuous glucose monitor for six months as of this writing. I have learned that when I eat a low-net-carb diet and my blood sugar starts to rise 10 to 30 points for no obvious reason, it is related to low insulin levels and it is time for me to eat more carbs. When I do that my blood sugar starts to drop quite dramatically.

Why does this happen?

One of the reasons, as we have seen, is that while your brain can run primarily on ketones and fats, it requires a certain amount of glucose to function properly. If you aren't providing glucose directly via your diet, your body cues the liver to produce it.

An alternate explanation is simply that your body is constantly adapting to ensure that you stay alive. During a long fast or extended periods of ketosis, your body is simply seeking to preserve its fat fuel. Remember that your cells can only use glucose or fat for fuel. When you are in a state of ketosis, the majority of your cellular energy is being derived from fat. When your body senses that food is scarce, your body is programmed to ensure that you have plenty of glucose to fuel functions.

As a result, your metabolism will adjust and slow down fat burning and increase gluconeogenesis by burning muscle instead of fat. Your body wants to hang on to your precious fat stores so you'll have access to them in the future. It's like hanging on to your longest-burning wood before a hard winter, especially when you don't know how cold it's going to get or when it will end.

Many of the clinicians I interviewed for this book who employ ketosis as a therapeutic strategy find that many of their patients lose muscle and gain fat after an extended time in ketosis. The amount of time is different for everyone, but genetics and mitochondrial differences seem to be the main determining factors. Those with hormonal challenges such as hypothyroidism can fall victim to this natural adaptation sooner than most. Common complaints during this phenomenon are lack of energy and weight gain that is difficult to lose.

VARIETY MAY BE THE KEY TO LIFE (NOT JUST THE SPICE)

I strongly believe that variety is an important biological principle. Using one form of exercise or diet exclusively for long periods of time is likely to cause unintended negative consequences no matter how useful the diet or exercise is. So after you have regained your ability to burn fat as your primary fuel, it is wise to integrate variety into your food plan.

So how long should you remain in nutritional ketosis?

The details of what types and amounts of dietary variety will work best are clearly individual and depend on how severely impaired your metabolism was prior to regaining fat-burning capability. My best advice is to continue the fat-burning protocol described in this book for as long as it takes your body to adapt to burning fat as your primary fuel. After that, you can maintain your benefits over the long term by using what I call feast-famine cycling, which I describe in detail below.

If you are battling cancer, consult with your clinician before making any dietary changes, but it may make sense to continue in fat-burning mode until that issue is resolved.

Before I outline feast-famine cycling, there are a few basic premises behind this theory that you should know:

- Reproduction is the number one priority of your innate intelligence. This can work for you or against you.

- Periodic major dietary shifts appear to spur different mechanisms that increase the odds of survival.[14]

- Ancient cultures strengthened their survival mechanisms naturally through seasonal dietary changes and environmental factors that impacted their food supply.[15]

- By continually requiring your metabolism to adapt to new dietary patterns, you increase hormone sensitivity, optimize growth and other important hormone levels, support brain function,[16] and strengthen your microbiome.

How to Use Feast-Famine Cycling

Once you have captured the ability to burn fat as your primary fuel, it is time to listen to your body and increase the flexibility in your diet. If done prudently, this will not impair your body's ability to burn fat.

The way I recommend doing this is through feast-famine cycling, which approximates the eating pattern of many of our ancient ancestors.

To the best of my knowledge there are no controlled studies that have examined the details of this strategy, although many in the bodybuilding community have used variations of this theme to optimize their performance.

One intriguing and very structured approach is one that Dr. Dan Pompa is using with his group of trained physicians who implement nutritional ketosis in their patients. They start with four or five days a week of Peak Fasting, one or two days a week of water fasting, and one or two days a week of feasting. If you do this you will need to carefully listen to your body and ideally follow your biometrics, such as your body fat percentage, weight, and ketone and glucose levels, to determine the best strategy for you.

A more holistic way of approaching this is to make seasonal shifts in your dietary intake, much like our ancestors were forced to do in response to environmental stressors, scarcity of food supply, or seasonal growing patterns. You could achieve this by spending your winters following MMT and maintaining a fat-burning state, implementing a four- to seven-day fast in the spring (consuming only water or bone broth), and then enjoying more veggies, berries, and lighter meats and fish during the summer.

Some do well switching between strict MMT and a more lenient, yet still whole foods–based, diet every three or four months because it offers more change and seems to reignite weight loss and reinvigorate motivation every time they shift their diet.

No matter which strategy you choose, I have found that regular variation in diet helps encourage long-term compliance to a healthy lifestyle because the change helps ward off feelings of frustration, deprivation, and even boredom with continually eating the same foods.

Conditions That Suggest You Need to Implement Diet Variety

- Not fat adapting (meaning not going into ketosis)
- Not losing weight
- Losing weight but losing lean tissue rather than fat and becoming "skinny fat"—which means you aren't technically overweight but you typically have low muscle tone, a concentration of fat around your abdomen, and poor markers of health, such as high blood sugar, elevated triglycerides, and high blood pressure
- Burning fat, but still experiencing low energy levels
- Hormone conditions, especially low thyroid

General Principles to Consider When Implementing

It makes sense to not restrict yourself to a rigid schedule, such as fasting every Friday. Remember: variety is key. So while you can use the 5-1-1 (Peak Fasting for five days, water fasting for one day, and feasting for one day) or the 4-2-1 approximate weekly ratio that

Dr. Pompa recommends, you could mix those days up throughout the month. The purpose of the feast days is to remind your body it's not starving, stop the breakdown of muscle, and reignite fat burning. The fast days boost your fat-burning efficiency.

During feasting you decrease the amount of fat you are consuming and increase healthy carbs and protein. Feasting does not give you permission to eat junk food! (Although small amounts on an irregular basis will likely not contribute to serious metabolic challenges, they also will not promote health.) Seek to increase your net-carb intake to 100 to 150 grams of healthy carbs like sweet potatoes, yams, berries, beets, or other root veggies. You may even tolerate small amounts of healthy grains, such as brown rice and quinoa.

You can also increase your protein intake, but it would be wise to synchronize this with the days you are strength training so you can take advantage of the anabolic boost that is provided by activating the mTOR pathway with additional protein. It would likely be wise to limit the increase to double your normal protein intake, but you can play around with increasing it up to three times.

It is important to remember that in no case should you have more than 25 grams of protein in one meal as that will likely exceed your body's ability to effectively use these amino acids and simply put an extra burden on your kidneys. So be careful to space your protein throughout the day.

During feast days it would still be best to follow the strategy of not eating for at least a few hours before bed, and if you do eat, have a light meal to optimize your mitochondrial function.

Treating Sleep Issues, Migraines, and Chronic Fatigue with Feast-Famine Cycling

Gina, one of my treasured home and garden assistants, is 48 years old. Although she has always led a healthy lifestyle and had loads of energy, she has had some health problems. When she was in her mid-30s, her lifelong sleep disorders—severe jaw clenching and night terrors—were taking a heavy toll on her health.

She went to a sleep disorder center, and the doctor who saw her prescribed Clonazepam (also known as Klonopin). When the medication didn't relieve her symptoms, the doctor increased her dosage and promised the cure was just on the horizon. Instead of a cure, Gina developed a toxic reaction.

Her symptoms were brutal and widespread, leading to years of misdiagnoses, including fibromyalgia, anxiety, depression, hypermania, post-traumatic stress disorder, dissociative stress disorder, severe adrenal insufficiency, adrenaline dominance, parasitic infection, blood infection, chronic fatigue syndrome, lupus, rheumatoid arthritis, and Lyme disease.

After years of struggling with swelling, chronic hives, migraines, excessive weight gain, heavy brain fog, insomnia, thick blood, extensive nerve issues, loss of taste and smell, and extreme exhaustion, she was frustrated, overweight, and tired.

I had her track her nutritional intake for a week and reviewed it with her. At that point we decided to implement the high-fat, low-carb, adequate-protein diet. The first two weeks were difficult, but after that she found that following the program became both very easy and very satisfying. "Being in a fat-burning state provided a fantastic rush of clarity and energy," Gina recalls. In addition, her weight dropped and some symptoms eased up a bit.

After about a year of eating this way, Gina plateaued. Though better than when she started, she still had many issues and her weight was still excessive, especially considering that she had an active, nonsedentary lifestyle. At that point, we revisited her diet. I had her log everything she ate on Cronometer to be aware of what she was eating and in what portions. We then implemented a hard-core strategy to reset her system.

She did a four-day water fast and then followed an extreme low-carb and low-protein diet—limiting herself to 5 grams of carbs and 5 grams of protein with unlimited good fats—for 23 more days. Gina shared that it was very difficult to stick with the plan, but she worked through it.

At that point, we moved her to 20 grams of carbs and 20 grams of protein, still with unlimited fats, for another 21 days. Needless to say, she found this easier and experienced further weight loss and a slow but consistent easing of her symptoms. Then she hit another plateau. At that point we implemented feast-famine cycling with four days of high fat (unlimited), low to moderate protein (20 grams) and low carbs (20 grams); one day of water fasting; and two days of higher carbs (100 to 150 grams), higher protein (50 grams), and not so much fat. I instructed her to play with the number of days, the frequency, and the order to find her sweet spot of both physical and mental health.

In the last three months Gina has lost 20 pounds. She states that she is feeling better than she has felt in the last decade. Her sleep is significantly better, her energy level is rising, the excessive swelling in her hands is dissipating, her migraines have dropped by 90 percent, her muscles no longer constantly burn in pain, she grinds her teeth less, her night terrors have decreased markedly in both intensity and number of occurrences, and her brain fog is lifting. She is a work in progress but is finally optimistic that she can take control and regain her health, her energy, her mental capacity, and her healthy weight goals.

CHAPTER 11

OTHER WAYS TO IMPROVE YOUR MITOCHONDRIAL HEALTH

Hands down, changing your diet is the single most powerful thing you can do to improve the health of your mitochondria. Fasting is a close second, so be sure to review Chapter 10 to find a way to introduce fasting into your life that works for you.

There are other complementary strategies you can use to support your mitochondria further. This chapter covers those tools.

A note about aging: mitochondrial biogenesis (the making of new mitochondria) typically declines with age, resulting in a lower volume of mitochondria. So the older you are, the more you stand to benefit from these additional strategies.

Grounding

Throughout this book, I've discussed how excessive ROS production and secondary free radicals that occur as a result of using glucose rather than fat as your primary fuel source will impair your mitochondrial function.

So far I've concentrated on reducing the threat of ROS damage by opting for healthy fat as your primary fuel because it burns cleaner and produces far fewer free radicals in the process.

But there is another side of the equation, which is to provide your body with surplus electrons to neutralize excessive free radicals. Grounding is a great way to achieve this protection. Grounding simply means connecting with the earth directly with either bare feet or in leather-soled shoes (which are conductive).

The earth's surface is electrically conductive and is maintained at a negative potential by a variety of factors:

- Solar wind entering the magnetosphere; ionospheric winds

- Thunderstorms

- Molten magnetite that rotates in the earth's core, which is a potent source of free electrons that escape to the earth's surface

So the surface of the earth is a large reservoir of free electrons, and being in direct contact with the ground helps transfer beneficial electrons to your body. Unfortunately, most people who live in the developed world never gain access to this abundant supply of electrons, because if they are walking on dirt, they are wearing shoes with synthetic rubber soles that insulate their feet from the ability to ground. Aside from its antioxidant effects, grounding has many other benefits,[1, 2] including:

- Helps diminish the effect of nonnative electromagnetic fields from electronic devices like cell phones, computers, and Wi-Fi

- Speeds wound healing

- Relieves pain
- Promotes better sleep
- Reduces inflammation
- Provides a general sense of well-being
- Improves heart rate variability

Medical infrared imaging shows that inflammation begins to subside within 30 minutes of grounding. Within 40 minutes, energy production increases, as do oxygen consumption, pulse rate, and respiratory rate.

Furthermore, grounding also helps calm your sympathetic nervous system, which in turn supports your heart rate variability and promotes homeostasis, or balance, in your autonomic nervous system. This is important because any time you improve your heart rate variability, you're improving your entire body and all its functions. Heart rate variability is a rarely discussed but is a potent marker of good overall health.

Simple Ways to Get Grounded

Many Americans spend most of their waking hours wearing shoes with rubber or plastic soles. These materials are very effective insulators, which is precisely why they're used to insulate electrical wires. Yet they also effectively disconnect you from the earth's natural electron flow. Wearing leather-soled shoes will allow you to stay grounded with the earth, as will walking barefoot, but you'll need to do so on the proper surface.

Good grounding surfaces include:

- Sand (beach)
- Grass (preferably moist)
- Bare soil
- Concrete and brick (as long as it's not painted or sealed)
- Ceramic tile

The following surfaces will *not* ground you:

- Asphalt
- Wood
- Rubber and plastic
- Vinyl
- Tar or tarmac

The ideal location for walking barefoot is the beach, close to or in the water, as seawater is a great conductor. A close second to the beach is a grassy area, especially if it's covered with dew, which is what you'll find if you walk early in the morning.

Even if you can't walk on the beach or on dewy grass, it's important to ground whenever possible with the sun shining directly on your skin, because it creates a biological circuit between the sun, you, and the earth in order to enhance your cellular energy production. Please see the next section for a detailed explanation of why this is so.

This is one of the reasons why I take a barefoot one- to three-hour walk on the beach nearly every day, as it helps me fulfill my movement requirements while also grounding me to the earth and providing me with the beneficial wavelengths that are virtually impossible to get if I spend all day indoors.

While moving is ideal, you don't need to be in motion in order to ground. For example, you could set up a chair outside and let your bare feet rest on the ground while you read your morning paper.

If you live in an urban area where there is no good and easy access to the ground, or simply can't get outside regularly for whatever reason, you can buy grounding pads and sheets that you plug into a grounded rod. You can purchase these on Amazon or at your local hardware store for about $10. You run the wire through a window or drill through the wall and fill the hole with silicone. This is the ideal way to ground indoors. You can plug into a grounded electrical circuit, although many are concerned about nonnative electromagnetic frequencies from dirty electricity being transferred into your body. Remember that grounding indoors is far inferior to outdoor grounding with the sun shining on your skin, for reasons I detail in the next section.

Sensible Sun Exposure

One of the most important strategies you can implement is to be outside in the sunshine every seasonally appropriate day with as much of your skin exposed as possible. If you've followed me for any length of time, you know that I am a major proponent of healthy sun exposure because it helps boost levels of vitamin D. What I am now beginning to see is that the healing power of sunshine goes beyond its role in vitamin D production.

This is so because in many ways we are similar to plants in that we are designed to collect all the wavelengths of solar radiation and use them to regulate and even fuel a number of very important physiological processes. And we are only beginning to recognize and understand all the ways sunshine affects us. This topic, also known as photobiology, fascinates me so much it will likely be the focus of my next book.

Sunshine is composed of all the wavelengths of light in a balanced form in the ideal proportion. It is what your ancient ancestors were regularly exposed to, and as a result your biology is optimized to receive nutrition from sunlight.

When you spend most of your time indoors, you deprive yourself of vital frequencies such as UV and infrared light that are typically not present in most artificial indoor light. Even in the daytime, windows tend to filter out many beneficial wavelengths.

Historically our ancient ancestors spent much if not most of their time outdoors and were grounded to the earth. A large part of the reason for sunlight's healing benefits is that it is a potent source of photons, which are an elementary particle of electromagnetic radiation that includes light. They can be both wave and particle, as Einstein deduced, and they are containers for energy. The reason the sun can produce electricity via solar panels is that its photons interact with atoms in the solar panel and knock out a few electrons from the atoms, creating electricity.

In some ways you are similar to a solar panel. When you are outside (preferably in direct contact to the earth so that you are grounded) and the sun is shining on your skin, a powerful chain reaction occurs that can then provide energy to improve your mitochondrial function. This chain reaction is particularly potent when you are grounded, as it helps create a circuit where the flow of energy through your body can be significantly improved.

This is especially true if you have sufficient levels of the omega-3 fatty acid DHA incorporated into your cellular and mitochondrial membranes. DHA is the only fat we know of that is capable of accepting the sun's photons and converting them to DC electric current. This is called the photoelectric effect, and Einstein received a Nobel Prize in 1921 for this discovery.

The current that is created helps structure the water in your cells in a process that makes water molecules better organized and thus better able to penetrate your cells. This provides for superior hydration and helps the water molecules store a charge that will provide fuel for your mitochondria.

One of the other functions of ultraviolet radiation is that it stimulates the production of nitric oxide in your skin, which can dilate blood vessels and shunt up to 60 percent of the blood flow to the surface of the skin, where the solar radiation can be more easily transferred to the blood.

It's ultraviolet B radiation that influences vitamin D production, but the other wavelengths provide important functions too. I'll discuss the power of red and infrared light next.

INFRARED SAUNA

To optimize this biological circuit I just described, it would be ideal to have several hours a day with sun exposure on your skin while grounded to the earth. Obviously this is impractical for most people, but if you are seriously debilitated from a health problem, you might be motivated to create the opportunity to implement an intervention like this.

It might involve making a change in your location to more of a tropical or subtropical environment. Combining such a move with MMT would likely result in a powerful synergy that could help reverse whatever health challenge you are currently struggling with.

Those without serious health challenges who are unable to spend significant time outside every day throughout the year would likely receive benefit from low-EMF, full-spectrum infrared sauna therapy.

Red and infrared light penetrate deeply into your tissues, delivering energy to your mitochondria, which use it to increase ATP production. In addition to this very important role in improving your mitochondrial function, an infrared sauna can also be very valuable in helping you remove toxins you have acquired throughout your lifetime.

It is my best guess that most everyone would benefit from regular sessions (two to three times a week) of infrared sauna therapy to remove stored toxins. I do these nearly every day when I am home.

If you are going to use an infrared sauna regularly, be sure you use one that has low EMF; most models emit high levels of non-native EMF. You can easily measure this by turning the sauna on and using an inexpensive electrical meter (like Trifield EMF meter) to measure the field inside the sauna. The level should be below 1 milligauss and preferably below 0.3.

Many companies advertise their saunas as full spectrum but in fact they are not. Most infrared saunas are far infrared, and while that is useful, especially for detox, it is incomplete. The near-infrared wavelengths, especially 800 to 850 nanometers, are what cytochrome c oxidase, the fourth protein in the electron transport chain in your mitochondria, resonates with. This is important if you hope to optimize your ATP and cellular energy production.

If you are purchasing a sauna, make sure the manufacturer supplies you with third-party analysis that shows you have levels of near infrared in the 800 to 850 nm range that are just as high as the far infrared. Most saunas have far-infrared levels that are 20 times higher than near infrared. So be careful and do your homework before making an important health investment like a low-EMF full-spectrum infrared sauna.

The heat from the sauna also has some additional metabolic benefits because exposing your body to heat helps activate genes that are important for optimizing heat-shock proteins inside your cells. This is important, as these proteins get damaged with time and need to be renewed. Accumulation of damaged HSPs can lead to plaque formation in your brain and/or vascular system, and heat stress helps prevent this adverse chain of events.

HSPs are also involved in longevity, so it's really good to have a lot of them. They're also important for preventing your skeletal muscle from atrophying because they protect proteins from being degraded.

Heat also promotes mitochondrial biogenesis because it is a stress that triggers the release of ROS, and ROS in this scenario call for making more mitochondria. To be clear, if your health is seriously compromised, it is essential to consult with your clinician before using sauna therapy.

ARTIFICIAL LIGHTING

Light engineers have done a magnificent job of producing energy-efficient lighting in the form of LEDs. They produce brilliant blue light that seems to replicate sunlight. But looks can be deceiving, and I was certainly fooled when I switched over to LED lighting around 2010.

What I failed to realize is that LEDs produce light that is very high in blue and low in red light. While blue light is not inherently dangerous, it is when taken out of its proper biological context. In fact, we are designed to have blue light exposure in the early-morning hours but not in the evening and nighttime hours. And the blue light we are designed to receive comes from sunlight, not LED bulbs.

Sunlight is perfectly balanced. It contains equal amounts of red and blue light and is also balanced with infrared, near-infrared, and ultraviolet light, further complementing its health benefits. When you are exposed to LEDs, the high concentration of blue light can cause some serious problems.

It is well known that blue light exposure after sunset can disrupt circadian rhythms and decrease natural melatonin production, which can increase your risk of cancer.[3] That is why wearing blue-blocking glasses after sunset is a profoundly useful strategy to limit this exposure.

Very few yet understand that this non-sunlight blue light exposure is also problematic during the day. Studies clearly show that blue exposure from LED or fluorescents increases ROS in the retina, but this is only problematic (i.e., potentially damage causing) when the blue light comes from an artificial source. This is especially true when you are indoors and have no access to natural light from a window. Blue light from sunlight is balanced by the red and infrared frequencies that are also present in sunlight, and these stimulate the repair and recovery pathways that help the retina and your body recover from blue light exposure.

Many studies show that exposure to blue light from LED lights contributes to macular degeneration, as blue light penetrates more deeply into the eye than UV light and can reach the retina, where the oval-shaped macula is located. Although if macular degeneration is caught early, its progress can be slowed, the vision loss it causes is typically irreversible and if left unchecked will become severe.

Macular degeneration is currently the most common cause of vision loss. My guess is that unless the message about the dangers of non-thermal artificial blue light from LEDs and fluorescents is spread to the public, there will likely be an epidemic of macular degeneration in the next decade or two. Some estimates project that 90 percent of our artificial light will come from LEDs by the year 2020.[4] While no one can dispute the energy savings gained from digital lighting, virtually no one is exploring the biological consequences of this shift. Once again we may be dealing with a massive dose of unintended consequences, substituting energy savings for vision loss.

To more clearly understand the danger blue light poses to your eyes, it's helpful to look to the color-rendering index (CRI). The CRI describes how a light source makes the color of an object appear to human eyes and how well subtle variations in color shades are revealed. Using a scale from 0 to 100, it indicates how accurate a "given" light source is at rendering color when compared to a "reference" light source.

The higher the CRI, the better the color rendering ability. Light sources with a CRI of 85 to 90 are considered good at color rendering. Light sources with a CRI of 90 or higher are excellent. Full sunlight has a CRI of 100.

Most incandescent bulbs have a CRI of 99, while most LED bulbs have CRI in the low 70s. While incandescent bulbs are "inefficient" because less than 5 percent of the energy they consume is used to produce visible light, the rest of the energy is converted to heat, another term for infrared light.

While we certainly can't use that "wasted" energy from the incandescent bulbs to see, it is a thermal source of lighting and produces a very similar wavelength distribution as sunlight. The "wasted" nonvisible wavelengths appear to have great biological value.

Many human studies need to be done to confirm the biological effects of LED light exposure, but that does not mean you need to wait decades for the result and suffer from this exposure until everyone agrees we need more balanced sources of light.

Additionally, LED lights are digital and as such flicker, or go on and off, at a very high frequency that may have some negative biological consequences. Conversely, incandescent lights are analog thermal light sources that are virtually identical to the light our ancestors used for millennia. As such, our biology is well adapted to them.

I believe there are some simple strategies you can now implement to protect your health from the blue light exposure that comes from LEDs.

Ideally, you should use as few lights as possible at night. Those you do use should be clear incandescents that do not have a coating to create whiter light. It would still be wise to wear blue-blocking glasses even with incandescents. It would be very wise to avoid the use of any LED lighting after sunset. Halogens are another acceptable form of incandescent lighting.

LED lighting during daylight hours is potentially less problematic, as the blue light is less likely to disrupt melatonin and circadian rhythm cycles. But be careful: if there is no outside light to balance the excessive blue light from the LEDs, it's best to wear blue-blocking glasses during the day too.

Although lighting is the primary sources of LED exposure, many fail to appreciate the dangers of their TV, desktop monitors, notebooks, tablets, and phones. The same cautions apply here. They are less problematic during the daytime but really should not be viewed without blue-blocking glasses after sunset.

Thankfully, the nighttime danger of blue light has finally begun to be appreciated, and the electronics industry offers a number of solutions. Apple launched Night Shift in iOS version 9, and Android version 6 has a blue light filter. For desktop monitors, there is a program called f.lux that will block out much of the blue light. But even better than f.lux is Iris, which is far easier to use and can provide much better blue light filtering; it can be obtained at http://iristech.co/iris-mini/. I use this application on all my computers to eliminate all blue light that f.lux is unable to do.

Remember that it is important to block the blue light to the lowest level while still being able to read the screen. In bright sunlight you won't be able to see the screen unless you don't block any of the blue light. This is fine, though: the red and other frequencies from the sunlight will block any dangers of blue light.

Also note that if you wake up before sunrise, using blue light–blocking glasses would be a wise strategy. Wear them until the sun rises. This will help maintain your very important circadian rhythm. This is especially important during the winter when there is not much daylight.

EXERCISE

Exercise is a proven method to improve the function of your existing mitochondria and stimulate the production of additional mitochondria through the process of mitochondrial biogenesis, which in turn provides even more ATP for your cells. Exercise increases mitochondrial biogenesis by activating peroxisome proliferator-activated receptor gamma coactivator (PGC-1alpha), a long mouthful of a name for the most important stimulus for mitochondrial biogenesis.

Exercise also activates a powerful signaling mechanism called adenosine monophosphate-activated protein kinase (AMPK), which promotes mitochondrial biogenesis via PGC-1alpha up-regulation and simultaneously triggers the destruction of existing defective mitochondria through mitophagy.

When you exercise, your body responds by creating more mitochondria to keep up with the cell's heightened energy requirement. When it comes to maintaining optimal biological functioning and good health, the more healthy mitochondria you have, the better off you'll be. Exercise is also a form of beneficial heat stress because it causes an elevation of your core temperature.

I am a true exercise devotee and have much more to say about the subject. Either visit fitness.mercola.com or search my site for my short book *Dr. Mercola's Guide to Optimal Fitness* for more practical information on how to incorporate more exercise and movement into your life.

COLD THERMOGENESIS

Cold thermogenesis is another stressor that is similar to heat stress in that it stimulates beneficial biological adaptations. Cold stress helps your body burn fat as its primary fuel because regular cold exposure increases your stores of brown fat—a particular type of fat that is far more effectively used for fuel than the more prevalent white fat. When you're exposed to cold, your brain increases production of norepinephrine and dopamine, both involved in focus and attention. These neurotransmitters also improve mood and alleviate pain, partly because they lower inflammation. You can increase norepinephrine twofold just by getting into 40-degree water for 20 seconds, or 57-degree water for a few minutes.

While best known as a neurotransmitter, norepinephrine also acts as a hormone. One of its functions is causing vasoconstriction, which helps your body conserve heat. Norepinephrine also acts as a signaling molecule to make more mitochondria in your fat tissue (your main energy reserves), and a by-product of energy production is heat.

This also helps prepare you for the next time you're exposed to cold. The more times you're exposed to cold, the more mitochondria you make in your fat cells and the better you can withstand lower temperatures.

So yes, you can become acclimated to colder temperatures with time. This is because that previous cold exposure has cued your fat to make more mitochondria. This means you are capable of burning more fat for fuel, the result of which is heat, and that heat makes it possible for you to tolerate colder conditions for a longer period of time.

Just as when you expose yourself to heat you make heat-shock protein, when exposing yourself to cold you also make a cold-shock protein known as RNA-binding motif 3, or RBM3, in your brain. Animal studies have shown that RBM3 can help ward off Alzheimer's disease,[5] suggesting that cold therapy can also have neuroprotective effects in addition to boosting your mitochondria, aiding in fat loss, and resolving leptin resistance.

There is one important caveat worth mentioning: When you're doing strengthening exercises, you generate ROS that help increase muscle mass. If you expose yourself to cold within the first hour after strength training, you suppress that beneficial process, so avoid doing cold immersion (such as a really cold shower or ice bath) immediately after strength training.

While sauna bathing and cold water immersion are generally safe, if you have any sort of medical condition, discuss it with your doctor beforehand, since both hot and cold put stress on your heart and cardiovascular system. Also, listen to your body. Individual tolerance for hot and cold temperatures varies widely, and if you push it too far you can harm yourself.

You can begin to implement cold thermogenesis by filling a small sink with ice water. Measure the water temperature so it stays between 50 and 55 degrees. Before you start, remove all makeup from your face and eat a high-fat meal. When you are ready, dunk your face in the water and hold it there as long as you can, gradually extending the duration until you are forced to remove your head from the water so you can take a breath.

From there, you can move on to taking cold showers and eventually work your way up to cold baths using multiple bags of ice. Any time you experience light-headedness or pale-pink to white skin, stop the treatment and try again another time for a shorter duration.

SUPPLEMENTS

Your mitochondria require many elements to function properly. You will get most of these from the foods on the MMT plan, but there are a few you might want to take in supplement form to ensure a more than adequate supply. These include:

Berberine

Berberine is a yellow alkaloid compound found in several different plants, including European barberry, goldenseal, goldthread, Oregon grape, phellodendron, and tree turmeric. It has antimicrobial, anti-inflammatory, and immune-enhancing properties and is effective against a wide range of bacteria, protozoa, and fungi. It can be used topically on cuts and other wounds, and it's perhaps most commonly used to treat gastrointestinal issues, including traveler's diarrhea and food poisoning.

To understand the true power of berberine—and why it now vies for a position as one of the most potent supplements anywhere—it's important to understand AMPK. Active components in berberine result in many of the same benefits as cleaning up your diet and exercising more, and they do so primarily by activating AMPK, one of the few nondrug compounds known to do so.

AMPK is an important nutrient-sensing pathway that is inversely associated with mTOR levels. So when you have high insulin, leptin, or IGF-1, it increases mTOR and correspondingly decreases AMPK. If done chronically, this is not good for your health. Conversely, when you have low insulin, IGF-1, and leptin levels, you inhibit mTOR and activate AMPK, which pushes your biology in the healthy direction.

AMPK also plays an important role in regulating metabolism by normalizing lipid, glucose, and energy imbalances as well as playing an active role in cellular repair and maintenance. When AMPK is activated, it helps you burn fats more effectively.

Berberine also boosts brown fat activity. Brown fat is a type of fat that *burns* energy instead of storing it. It is loaded with mitochondria, which is why it is brown, and those mitochondria are responsible for converting fat directly to energy to produce heat.

Berberine also:

- Acts as a powerful antioxidant, scavenging free radicals

- Stimulates the clearance of glucose from your bloodstream

- Inhibits glucose production in your liver

- Improves insulin sensitivity

- Displays significant anticancer activity against multiple cancer cell types in many signaling network pathways

Berberine has a short half-life, so if you're interested in using this supplement, you generally need to take it three times a day to keep blood levels stable. Many studies have looked at dosages of 900 to 1,500 mg per day, which you could break down into 300 to 500 mg three times a day before meals.

Ubiquinol

Ubiquinol is the fully reduced version of coenzyme Q10 (CoQ10). It is an important participant in reactions that occur in the five cytochromes in the electron transport chain within your mitochondria. There, it facilitates the conversion of energy substrates and oxygen into energy.

Ubiquinol is one of the few fat-soluble antioxidants, meaning it works in the fat portions of your body, such as your cell membranes, to mop up ROS—those potentially harmful by-products of the metabolic process. Taking this supplement can protect your mitochondrial membranes from oxidative damage.

Dosing requirements vary depending on your individual situation and needs, but as a general rule, the sicker you are, the more you'll need to take. If you're severely ill, 600 mg per day may be appropriate. But if you're just starting out with ubiquinol, begin with 200 to 300 mg per day.

Within three weeks your plasma level will typically plateau to its optimum point. After that, you can reduce your dosage to 100 mg per day, a reasonable maintenance dose. This amount is typically sufficient for healthy people. If you have an active lifestyle, exercise a lot, or are under a lot of stress due to your job or life in general, you may want to increase your dose to 200 to 300 mg per day.

If you're on a statin drug—and more than one in four American adults over the age of 40 are—you must take at least 100 to 200 mg of ubiquinol per day. This is because statins work by inhibiting the enzyme HMG-CoA reductase, which not only facilitates your body's endogenous production of cholesterol, but also impairs the production of CoQ10, the precursor of ubiquinol. The subsequent depletion can have very severe consequences.

Ideally, you'll want to work with your physician to determine your best dose. Your doctor can do a blood test to measure your CoQ10 levels, or do an organic acid test, which would tell you whether your dose is high enough to keep you within a healthy range.

One note of caution about statins and MMT: If you're on statins and following MMT, it's important to know that HMG-CoA reductase, the enzyme that statins reduce, also plays a role in the production of ketones. So when you're taking a statin drug, you also severely and profoundly interfere with your liver's ability to make ketones. Even if you start taking ubiquinol, you still have to address the fact that your ability to convert fats to ketones is seriously impaired. If you are dedicated to trying MMT, you may want to work with your doctor to get off statins.

Another important note: Because both are mitochondrial antioxidants, ubiquinol and CoQ10 may work against chemotherapy drugs, so please be aware of this if you are seeking to treat cancer with nutritional ketosis. The increased activity of CoQ10 within the electron transport chain may increase cancer cell mitochondrial energy production, contributing to the increased likelihood of inducing intrinsic recycling (apoptosis) of cancer cells. The anticancer intervention is to avoid oral antioxidants vitamin C, most forms of vitamin E, most forms of selenium, and importantly, N-acetyl-cysteine, as adding this antioxidant produces increased cancer cell mitochondrial strength and confers survival advantage to the cancer cell mitochondria. However, as I mentioned in chapter 1, high dose IV vitamin C or oral liposomal C is used by many integrative cancer physicians to kill cancer cells, so please consult with your physician to customize this recommendation for your specific circumstances.

Strategies for mitochondria management in patients with cancer are fundamentally different from strategies for mitochondria management in patients with other chronic diseases. Treatment that is good for diseased non–cancer cell mitochondria can be very dangerous for a patient with cancer because that same treatment can make the cancer cells stronger and resistant to being harmed by specific anticancer treatments.

This is a serious problem among natural medicine practitioners who unknowingly administer cancer-strengthening antioxidants to patients with cancer out of lack of understanding of the molecular biology of cancer cell mitochondria compared to other cells' mitochondria.

Magnesium

Magnesium is a mineral every organ in your body needs, especially your heart, muscles, and kidneys, yet the majority of us are deficient in this vital nutrient and don't even know it. By some estimates, up to 80 percent of Americans are not getting enough magnesium and may be deficient. This is why magnesium deficiency has been dubbed the "invisible deficiency."

A century ago, people received an estimated 500 mg of magnesium from their diet courtesy of the nutrient-rich soil in which food was grown. Today, estimates suggest we're only getting 150 to 300 mg a day from our food. The RDA is around 310 to 420 mg depending on your age and sex, although some researchers believe we may need as much as 600 to 900 mg/day for optimal health.

Magnesium is an important component of success with MMT because it participates in the process of energy creation by activating ATP. Thus, magnesium is vital for the optimization of your mitochondria.

If you exhibit any early signs of magnesium deficiency such as "charley horses," headaches, loss of appetite, nausea and vomiting, fatigue, or weakness, consider adding magnesium as a supplement. My personal preference is magnesium threonate because it appears to be most effective at penetrating cell membranes, including mitochondrial membranes, which can help boost your energy level. It also crosses your blood-brain barrier and may help improve circulation and memory.

Carnitine

L-carnitine, which is derived from amino acids, is found in red meat, eggs, and other MMT-friendly foods. Carnitine shuttles long-chain fats across your mitochondrial membranes so they can be oxidized for energy. When you burn fat for fuel, as MMT will help you do, you will use up more carnitine than you do when you burn glucose for fuel, so you may become temporarily deficient. It can take a while for your carnitine levels to stabilize at an appropriate level, which they will typically do on MMT. To be clear, your mitochondria will still be able to use ketones and medium-chain fats, but if your carnitine level is low it will be more of a challenge to oxidize longer-chain fats.

As I discussed concerning carnitine and its role in Chapter 8, the best way to determine your carnitine level is with a blood test. If the results show that your levels are indeed low and you are experiencing symptoms such as low energy or fatigue, or if you are not producing enough ketones to fully adapt to fat burning, you may want to supplement with carnitine. If you do supplement, you may only need to do so for a while with 500 or 1,500 mg per day; your body can make its own carnitine, and it just may take some time for it to adjust this internal balance.

Keep in mind that there is mixed evidence on whether supplemental carnitine may contribute to cancer progression, so if you have cancer, even if your levels are low, you may want to hold off on supplementing.

Structured Water

A source of clean water is one of the most important factors to optimize your health. Considering that it is so ubiquitous, it is surprising that water hasn't received more scientific analysis.

Dr. Gerald Pollack is a biophysicist at the University of Washington and is one of the leaders in analyzing how water powers our biology. He has written a book called *The Fourth Phase of Water*, which I highly recommend for anyone seeking to understand more about the magnificent function and role that water plays in biology and our health.

Pollack details on how water can be transformed into structured water (the fourth phase of water), which he calls EZ (exclusion zone) water. EZ is the scientific term for what physically happens to water once it is transformed into structured water, which actually has a different chemical structure than tap water, H_2O. Structured water has different hydrogen bonding and is actually H_3O.

One of the best ways you can facilitate this process of helping your body create more intracellular structured water is to make certain that you have regular exposure to sunlight on your skin. Sunlight contains about 40 percent infrared (especially near-infrared) light, which helps catalyze the transformation of cellular water into structured water. You can also achieve this through regular use of a low-EMF infrared sauna, which will also help your body release toxins stored in your fat.

If for any reason you are unable to regularly access sunlight or a low-EMF, full-spectrum infrared sauna, it would be helpful to drink structured water that is created by pressure, movement (particularly vortices), or exposure to cold temperatures, beneficial electromagnetic fields, unipolar static magnetic fields, or infrared or UV light. As such, the best ways to obtain it are from:

- Deep natural springs (use findaspring.com to find one near you)

- Cooling it to about 39 degrees Fahrenheit (about 4 degrees centigrade)

- Stirring the water with a spoon in a circular jar to create a vortex, or purchasing a vortex machine for this purpose

- Eating or juicing raw vegetables (as vegetables are loaded with structured water but tend to lose it once they are cooked or heated)

IN CONCLUSION

In summary, it's time to reverse the demonization of healthy fats and our reliance on refined and processed carbohydrates as the bulk of our diet that has caused most of us to lose the ability to burn fat as our primary fuel.

Teaching your body to relearn how to burn fat as your primary fuel is one of the most important and foundational strategies you can implement to lose weight, ease inflammation, relieve troubling symptoms, and prevent chronic diseases.

I strongly encourage you to be kind to your body and let it start burning the fuel it needs to get you to better health. Persevere and you will be rewarded and pleasantly surprised to see how your food cravings decease and your energy level improves.

Remember, though, that improving mitochondrial function is an evolving science. It will likely be many years before this approach is widely adopted. If you want to keep deepening your understanding of how to take care of your mitochondria and continue to improve your health even before the science has fully solidified around this subject, I have two suggestions for you:

- Seek the assistance of professionally trained and certified professionals who can consult with you and help you implement the program successfully. They will also help you develop a deeper understanding of the best way to give your body the fuel it needs to survive. Find one at www.nutritionspecialists.org.

- Stay current on the latest research and subsequent refinements to MMT at my website, www.mercola.com. I regularly review the published studies on this topic, and if any major developments or changes to the program that I describe in this book occur, I will outline them there. There is never a charge to review any of these articles and you can always use the search tab at the top of every page on the site to find out details on any health topic.

I want to congratulate you on making it through this book. I know it is science-heavy and that the dietary changes I suggest may at first seem daunting, but I hope that you will find it a useful and valuable guide to a brighter health future. I wish you the best in your efforts to take control of your health.

RESOURCES

BOOKS

The Art and Science of Low Carbohydrate Living, by Stephen D. Phinney and Jeff S. Volek

The Art and Science of Low Carbohydrate Performance, by Stephen D. Phinney and Jeff S. Volek

The Big Fat Surprise: Why Butter, Meat and Cheese Belong in a Healthy Diet, by Nina Teicholz

Cancer as a Metabolic Disease: On the Origin, Management, and Prevention of Cancer, by Dr. Thomas Seyfried, professor of biology at Boston College. You can learn more about the keto research conducted at Dr. Seyfried's lab on his website: http://www.bc.edu/schools/cas/biology/facadmin/seyfried.html.

The Complete Guide to Fasting: Heal Your Body By Intermittent, Alternate-Day, and Extended Fasting, by Jimmy Moore and Dr. Jason Fung

Doctoring Data: How to Sort Out Medical Advice from Medical Nonsense, by Dr. Malcolm Kendrick

Dumping Iron: How to Ditch This Secret Killer and Reclaim Your Health, by P. D. Mangan

Good Calories, Bad Calories: Fats, Carbs, and the Controversial Science of Diet and Health, by Gary Taubes

Grain Brain: The Surprising Truth About Wheat, Carbs, and Sugar—Your Brain's Silent Killers, by David Perlmutter, M.D., and Kristin Loberg

Keto Clarity: Your Definitive Guide to the Benefits of a Low-Carb, High-Fat Diet, by Jimmy Moore and Dr. Eric Westman

Keto for Cancer: The Ketogenic Diet as a Targeted Nutritional Strategy, A Guide for Patients and Practitioners based on the Metabolic Theory of Cancer, by Miriam Kalamian

Power, Sex, Suicide: Mitochondria and the Meaning of Life, by Nick Lane

The Obesity Code: Unlocking the Secrets of Weight Loss, by Dr. Jason Fung and Timothy Noakes

The Obesity Epidemic: What Caused It? How Can We Stop It? by Zoë Harcombe

Tripping over the Truth: How the Metabolic Theory of Cancer Is Overturning One of Medicine's Most Entrenched Paradigms, by Travis Christofferson

COOKBOOKS

200 Low-Carb, High-Fat Recipes: Easy Recipes to Jumpstart Your Low-Carb Weight Loss by Dana Carpender takes a very straightforward approach to incorporating more fat into your meals. Take note, though, that this author is not concerned about food quality. In other words, there's no mention of pasture raised versus CAFO or raw versus cooked. Still, the book is a practical resource, especially for those new to any kind of whole-food cooking.

The Ketogenic Cookbook: Nutritious Low-Carb, High-Fat Paleo Meals to Heal Your Body by Jimmy Moore and Maria Emmerich is an elegant take on high-fat gourmet, beautifully illustrated throughout. This is more special-occasion cooking than everyday, but is great for the foodies out there who fear monotony.

The Ketogenic Kitchen: Low carb. High fat. Extraordinary Health by Patricia Daly and Domini Kemp—both cancer survivors who have woven their story, as well as many cancer-fighting tips, into the book. Includes meal plans and recipes that may help those new to low-carb, high-fat cooking.

ONLINE RESOURCES

The Charlie Foundation for Ketogenic Therapies was founded to provide information, advocacy, and support for families with children suffering from intractable epilepsy. Over the years, it has expanded its mission to include use of the diet for cancer, autism, ALS, Parkinson's disease and Alzheimer's disease, and traumatic brain injury. It is a clearinghouse of scientific research, recipes, and products related to the therapeutic benefits of a ketogenic diet. http://www.charliefoundation.org/.

Cronometer, a free online tool that you can use to customize your MMT plan. Track food intake, add biometrics, and record exercise, then see at a glance if you are meeting your targets for macronutrient distribution, nutrient intake, and other parameters you wish to track. Cronometer is also available as an app, making it convenient for you to log your foods on the go. I am thrilled to have been able to collaborate with the founders to create a custom "Mercola" version of the software that's designed to support your efforts. You can find it here: http://www.cronometer.com/mercola.

Dietary Therapies, the website of Miriam Kalamian, Ed.M., M.S., C.N.S., nutrition consultant and educator who specializes in the ketogenic diet for cancer. She offers a book on her website that you can use as a guide to implementation. http://www.dietarytherapies.com/.

Ketogenic Diet Resource, the website of Ellen Davis, M.S. This site is particularly helpful for its general and condition-specific info as well as high-fat, moderate-protein, and low-carb food plans and recipes (although you may need to modify them because they may be too high in protein for you, depending on your lean body mass, so please keep that in mind). http://www.ketogenic-diet-resource.com.

KetoNutrition: Practical Information on Ketogenic Diets and Metabolic Therapies, the blog of top keto researcher Dominic D'Agostino, associate professor in the Department of Molecular Pharmacology and Physiology in the Morsani College of Medicine at the University of South Florida: http://ketonutrition.blogspot.com/ and http://ketonutrition.org/.

"Insulin and Its Metabolic Effects," a talk by Dr. Ron Rosedale. To view the transcript, go to: http://articles.mercola.com/sites/articles/archive/2001/07/14/insulin-part-one.aspx.

KetoDiet Blog, the blog of Martina Slajerova, author of *The KetoDiet Cookbook* and *Sweet and Savory Fat Bombs*—a great source of free, high-fat, low-carb recipes: http://www.ketodietapp.com/blog/.

Mercola.com, my own website where I publish articles daily on the latest research findings and updates in my own thinking and recommendations: www.mercola.com.

"Reconsidering the Role of Mitochondria in Aging," a 2015 research paper published in the *Journals of Gerontology: Medical Sciences,* is the best article I reviewed for this book and is available for free download at PubMed.gov (the National Institutes of Health's clearinghouse of scientific studies; you can find it by searching for "PMID: 25995290"). I did not dive deep into molecular pathways in this book, as it not written for professionals, but if you have extensive biochemical and mitochondrial education I would strongly encourage you to download this study. At the time of this writing, I have read it four times and learn something new with every read.

Ruled.me, a website with recipes and ketogenic high-fat food plans that also has an active forum: http://www.ruled.me.

SUPPLIES

Abbott Precision Xtra or Freestyle Optium Neo Blood Glucose and Ketone Monitoring Systems, meters that use test strips (which are typically sold separately) to measure beta-hydroxybutyrate and glucose in the blood—they may be called by another name outside of the U.S.

Bayer Contour Glucose Monitoring System, the most economical way to test blood glucose levels.

Bayer Ketostix, urine test strips to detect acetoacetate ketone bodies in the urine—best used in the first few months of the diet.

EatSmart Precision GetFit Digital Body Fat Scale, a bathroom scale that uses bioimpedance to assess your body fat percentage.

Ketonix Breath Ketone Analyzer, measures levels of acetone ketone bodies in the breath—particularly useful for athletes (https://www.ketonix.com).

Pure Power Mitomix Bars: These bars, which took 17 revisions to perfect, provide a high level of nutrients, great taste, and an MMT-friendly macronutrient ratio in a convenient grab-and-go package. They contain almond butter, psyllium, coconut, pumpkin seeds, macadamia nuts, cocoa powder, chia seeds, hemp seeds, coconut butter, cocoa powder, erythritol, and stevia in a chocolate coating (http://shop.mercola.com).

Skulpt Aim or Skulpt Chisel, electrical impedance myography (EIM) device to measure your body fat percentage.

APPENDIX A

From Pimples to Heart Disease: How Mitochondrial Metabolic Therapy Helps Many Diseases

Healing your mitochondria happens on the cellular level, but the benefits ripple throughout the body to include all aspects of your health—perhaps most dramatically the chronic diseases or conditions that may be threatening your quality of life.

The science community has recognized that a high-fat, ketogenic diet is beneficial for epilepsy since the 1920s. But it has been a slower road for research to assess the possible benefits of such a diet on a whole host of other conditions. Here is a roundup of the latest research on the long list of ailments that a fat-burning diet can help treat, if not outright reverse.

ACNE

Nearly 85 percent of people have acne at some point in their lives, making acne the most common skin disorder in the U.S.[1] While acne typically begins during puberty, it's not limited to adolescents and may impact any age group, even those in their 50s and beyond.

While not physically dangerous, acne can take a considerable psychological toll on its sufferers. Some of those afflicted become so self-conscious and embarrassed that their professional and personal lives suffer, leading to alienation, depression, and social withdrawal.

Many mistakenly believe acne is mostly an aesthetic problem, but it is actually a sign of a deeper imbalance in your system, often originating in your gut. Most physicians miss this connection entirely, instead prescribing acne drugs and other topical treatments.

Americans spend more than $2.2 billion every year on acne treatments, including prescription and over-the-counter products,[2] but many of these products will prove to be useless if you ignore the foundational cause of most acne: improper diet.

Diets high in sugar and refined carbohydrates are one of the primary causes of acne. In fact, acne is much less of a problem in non-Westernized societies, where refined carbohydrates and sugar are consumed in much lower amounts.[3]

The link between carbs and acne exists because grains, high-net-carb vegetables, fruits, and sugar/fructose all cause a surge of insulin and insulin-like growth factor 1 (IGF-1) in your body. Excess protein will also increase IGF-1. This can lead to an excess of male hormones, like testosterone, which cause your pores to secrete sebum, a greasy substance that attracts acne-promoting bacteria. IGF-1 also causes skin cells known as keratinocytes to multiply, a process that is also associated with acne.

Additionally, these very same foods—refined carbs—also increase inflammation in your body, which may trigger or exacerbate acne.

There is plenty of good evidence that changing your diet can result in improvements in acne. Most of the research does not look at high-fat diets but instead points to the benefits of eating a low-glycemic diet. Glycemic index refers to a food's ability to increase levels of blood sugars, so foods that are higher in carbs than in fiber (which helps stabilize blood sugar) also have a higher glycemic index. So although these studies aren't a total indicator of a high-fat diet's effect on acne, the MMT diet is also low glycemic, so there are strong parallels.

A 2007 study published in the *American Journal of Clinical Nutrition* found that young men (ages 15 to 25) with acne problems who were placed on low-glycemic diets for 12 weeks—in other words, diets low in the type of carbs that raise glucose and insulin— showed significant improvements in acne and insulin sensitivity.[4] A 2012 controlled randomized study by Korean researchers found that acne patients who followed a low-glycemic diet for 10 weeks experienced a significant reduction in inflammation and number of lesions.[5] And a 2014 review published by researchers at the State University of New York Downstate Medical Center examined evidence of a link between refined carbohydrate consumption and acne, concluding that dermatologists should counsel their acne patients to avoid high-glycemic (i.e., high-carb) foods,[6] which following the high-fat diet helps you do naturally, and without feelings of deprivation.

ALZHEIMER'S DISEASE

As of 2015, 5.3 million Americans had been diagnosed with Alzheimer's disease,[7] and that number has only steadily risen since then; Alzheimer's diagnoses are projected to triple by 2050.[8] Over half a million Americans die from the disease each year, making it the third leading cause of death in the U.S., right behind heart disease and cancer.[9]

Mounting research suggests that our modern diet is playing a significant role in the skyrocketing prevalence of Alzheimer's. Processed foods tend to be nearly devoid of healthy fat while loaded with refined sugars: a pernicious combination for mitochondrial function. As I discussed in the "mental clarity" section of Chapter 2, Alzheimer's has been considered "type 3 diabetes" since 2005, when researchers found that diabetics have a doubled risk of developing Alzheimer's disease.

Since then, researchers have begun to discover how insulin resistance and Alzheimer's are intricately linked. Insulin receptors are present throughout your brain, and play a role in learning and memory as well as the regulation of food intake and body weight.

When insulin signaling goes awry, it paves the way for cognitive decline and the development of Alzheimer's in two ways: First, it enhances key signaling molecules that, when stimulated, lead to the development of proteins that contribute to the plaques and tangles that occur in the brain and are hallmarks of the disease.[10] The other way doesn't initiate in the brain, but rather in the liver, which in the presence of insulin resistance produces toxic fats known as ceramides that then cross the blood-brain barrier and go on to cause insulin resistance, oxidative stress, inflammation, and cell death in the brain.[11]

Tying diet specifically to Alzheimer's is research from the Mayo Clinic published in 2012, which revealed that diets rich in carbohydrates are associated with an 89 percent increased risk for dementia, while high-fat diets are associated with a 44 percent reduced risk.[12]

MMT has great potential to support healthy brain function because it improves insulin receptor sensitivity that in turn improves overall metabolic signaling. It also catalyzes your body to burn fat for fuel, thereby radically increasing the amount of clean-burning ketones your body produces for fuel. It also lessens chronic inflammation and moderates high blood glucose levels, both of which are associated with Alzheimer's.

There have been a handful of studies on the effects of a functional food called Axona, which is made up of medium-chain triglycerides (MCTs)—saturated fats similar to those found in coconuts. A 2009 randomized, double-blind, and controlled study (considered the gold standard in research) found that Axona made a significant improvement in the cognitive function of patients with Alzheimer's disease when compared to placebo.[13] It's important to note that even though exogenous ketones can be useful and likely are highly beneficial for Alzheimer's disease, the first step is to get your body to make its own ketones.

Another avenue by which a high-fat diet could mitigate risk factors for Alzheimer's disease is by improving mitochondrial health. Brain images of living Alzheimer's patients and postmortem analyses have shown that impaired mitochondria accompany the disease.[14] Because MMT protects mitochondria from oxidative damage, it likely has a protective effect against Alzheimer's.

Fasting, which I covered in Chapter 10, further promotes MMT's beneficial effect on Alzheimer's disease because it can accelerate the breakdown of the amyloid plaques, or protein fragments, that are one of the hallmark brain abnormalities of Alzheimer's. When you keep your protein and net-carb levels low, you increase your brain's ability to remove and recycle these damaging protein fragments.

While the science is still evolving regarding the direct correlation between a high-fat diet and Alzheimer's disease, because there is no known way to reverse the disease once it is detected, prevention is key, and MMT has all the hallmarks of being an effective defense. Better yet, it is one that is 100 percent within your personal control—a key factor that Alzheimer's disease rapidly erodes once it sets in.

ARTHRITIS

More than 21 million Americans have trouble climbing stairs, getting dressed, and staying active due to arthritis, and that number is up from 19 million just a few years back. If you have osteoarthritis, the cartilage within your joints is undergoing progressive damage, and there is typically a reduction in the amount of synovial fluid that keeps your joints lubricated and cushioned. Osteoarthritis also has an inflammatory component.

By 2040, an estimated 78 million Americans over the age of 18 are expected to be diagnosed with osteoarthritis, with more than half of the new cases in people as young as 45 to 64 years.[15]

Why are so many young people suffering from this painful degenerative joint disease, which has historically been associated with wear and tear and joint deterioration that occur over a lifetime?

Rising rates of overweight and obesity likely play a role. Arthritis rates are more than twice as high in obese people as those who are normal weight, because the extra weight puts more pressure on their joints and increases inflammation in their bodies.

If you are one of the millions struggling with osteoarthritis, or want to avoid becoming one of that number, changing your diet is one of the simplest and most powerful steps you can take.

There is plenty of research showing that improving your omega-6 to omega-3 ratio—an integral part of MMT—has exciting potential to prevent and treat arthritis. According to a 2011 animal study, a diet enriched with omega-3 fats reduced the majority of disease indicators[16] among guinea pigs engineered to develop osteoarthritis. This included both cartilage and subchondral bone changes, and the lead researcher noted that the evidence was strong that omega-3 fats may help prevent the disease and also slow its progression in those already diagnosed. A 2013 study published in the journal *Cartilage* also showed that omega-6 oils, when injected into cartilage cells, provoked an inflammatory response, where monounsaturated and saturated fats appeared to inhibit cartilage destruction.[17]

A high-fat, ketogenic diet in particular has also been shown to reduce pain and inflammation in animal studies.[18, 19] Meaning that adopting a healthy high-fat diet (which includes eating more omega-3 fats and fewer omega-6s) is a viable and very promising avenue to pursue in the relief of the pain and disability that can be brought on by osteoarthritis. As an added benefit, you stand to lose some of the excess weight that may be contributing to your discomfort and keeping you from being physically active.

CARDIOVASCULAR DISEASE

Even though the death rate from cardiovascular diseases—which includes heart attacks and stroke—declined by 29 percent between 2001 and 2010, it's still the number one cause of death in the U.S., despite advances in medical technology that should have radically reduced the rate. According to the U.S. Centers for Disease Control and Prevention (CDC), about 800,000 Americans die from cardiovascular disease annually.[20]

A quarter of these deaths—or about 200,000—could be prevented through simple lifestyle changes, and more than half (6 out of 10) of the preventable heart disease and stroke deaths occur in people under the age of 65.

If you want to understand the causes of heart disease, you have to look at how your arteries incur damage, and what factors contribute to blood clotting. Contrary to popular belief, there's no fat (cholesterol) "clogging the pipe" at all.

Total cholesterol will tell you virtually nothing about your disease risk (unless it's exceptionally elevated, above 330 or so, which would be suggestive of familial hypercholesterolemia— about the only circumstance in which a cholesterol-lowering drug would be appropriate, in my opinion). Two ratios that are far better indicators of heart disease risk are:

- **Your HDL-to-total-cholesterol ratio:** The higher this number the better as a low HDL ratio is a very potent heart disease risk factor. Just divide your HDL level by your total cholesterol. This percentage should ideally be above 24 percent. Below 10 percent, it's a significant indicator of risk for heart disease.

- **Your triglyceride-to-HDL ratios:** This ratio should ideally be below 2.

Additional risk factors for heart disease include:

- **Your fasting insulin level:** Any meal or snack high in carbohydrates like fructose and refined grains generates a rapid rise in blood glucose and then insulin to compensate for the rise in blood sugar. The insulin released from eating too many carbs promotes fat storage and makes it more difficult for your body to shed excess weight; and excess fat, particularly around your belly, is one of the major contributors to heart disease. One typically requires a physician's lab order for this test but it is relatively inexpensive even if you have to pay for it yourself.

- **Your fasting blood sugar level:** Studies have shown that people with a fasting blood sugar level of 100 to 125 mg/dl had a nearly 300 percent higher risk of having coronary heart disease than people with a level below 79 mg/dl.[21] I personally believe that you should make the changes needed to get your fasting blood sugar below 80, and this is easily monitored at home using a blood glucose meter (see Chapter 6 for more information on how to do this).

- **Your iron level:** Iron can be a very potent driver of oxidative stress, so if you have excess iron levels you can damage your blood vessels and increase your risk of heart disease. Iron levels can be monitored by testing blood levels of ferritin; ideally, your level should be between 60 and 80 ng/nl. For information on this test and others that will help you monitor your iron levels, see Chapter 4.

In a nutshell, preventing cardiovascular disease involves *reducing chronic inflammation* in your body, and a proper diet is an absolute cornerstone here. Although saturated fat has taken the blame for causing heart disease for the last several decades, even mainstream medicine is coming to the realization that the primary culprit in heart disease is *sugar consumption.*

A 2015 study published in the *Journal of the American Medical Association* concluded that there's "a significant relationship between added sugar consumption and increased risk for cardiovascular disease mortality." The 15-year study, which included data for 31,000 Americans, found that those who consumed 25 percent or more of their daily calories as added sugars were more than twice as likely to die from heart disease as those who got less than 10 percent of their calories from sugar. On the whole, the odds of dying from heart disease rose in tandem with the percentage of added sugar in the diet regardless of the age, sex, physical activity level, and body mass index.[22]

A 2014 study came to very similar conclusions. Here, those who consumed the most sugar—about 25 percent of their daily calories—were twice as likely to die from heart disease as those who limited their sugar intake to 7 percent of their total calories.[23]

A high-fat diet dramatically reduces the amount of sugar you consume, and it mitigates risk factors for cardiovascular disease in other important ways that are related to insulin. As Dr. Rosedale explains, insulin stores magnesium. If your cells become resistant to insulin, magnesium passes out of your body through your urine rather than getting stored in your cells.

Several meta-analyses have confirmed a high-fat diet's role in reducing multiple risk factors for cardiovascular disease. One study, published in the *Journal of the Academy of Nutrition and Dietetics* in 2013, looked at the differing effects of high-fat diets versus low-fat diets on blood lipid levels. It included 32 studies and found that high-fat diets resulted in significantly greater improvements in reductions of total cholesterol, LDL cholesterol, and triglycerides and beneficial increases in HDL cholesterol.[24]

In regard to stroke, a 2012 review of animal studies published in the *Journal of Neurochemistry*[25] found that both a ketogenic diet and the supplementation of ketone bodies were protective in ischemic stroke (due to a blocked artery) and had neuroprotective benefits after a stroke occurred. As the researchers stated, there was a "notable improvement in mitochondrial function, a decrease in inflammation, and an increase in expression of neurotrophins such as BDNF" in animals in a ketogenic state.

Seizure Disorder

In the U.S., seizure disorder affects an estimated 4.3 million adults and nearly 750,000 children below the age of 17.[26] It's a chronic neurological condition characterized by recurring seizures, which can have a significant impact on a person's quality of life, given the heightened risk of accidents and injuries.

Standard treatment for epilepsy includes antiepileptic drugs, which tends to control the problem for 60 to 65 percent of patients—although antiseizure drugs increase the risk of suicidal thoughts and behaviors and are associated with memory loss and hair loss. For the remaining 35 to 40 percent of epilepsy patients, the drugs don't work—but oftentimes a ketogenic diet *will*.

The high-fat diet was first recognized in the 1920s[27] as the best option in the treatment of seizure disorder until the introduction of Dilantin, which, as is the case with other antiseizure medications, often fails to control seizures. There's even a ketogenic diet special interest group at the American Epilepsy Society. It was organized by Dr. Thomas Seyfried, who today is one of the leading academic researchers investigating the use of the ketogenic diet as a treatment for cancer.

Due to his and other research, as well as advocacy efforts of The Charlie Foundation for Ketogenic Therapies, the ketogenic diet is widely accepted as a dietary therapy for the management of refractory (drug-resistant) seizures, especially in children.

A 2016 Cochrane Review[28] that evaluated seven randomized controlled studies on children with seizures found that the high-fat classic ketogenic diet (with 90 percent of calories from fat) resulted in reported rates of freedom from seizures as high as 55 percent and of a reduction in seizure frequency as high as 85 percent after three months. For the Modified Atkins Diet, the studies reported seizure freedom rates of only 10 percent and seizure reduction rates at just 60 percent, suggesting that the higher-fat classic diet yielded significantly better results.

The researchers concluded, "For people who have medically intractable epilepsy or people who are not suitable for surgical intervention, a KD remains a valid option."

FIBROMYALGIA, CHRONIC FATIGUE SYNDROME, AND CHRONIC PAIN

When I started my medical practice over three decades ago, fibromyalgia was so commonly missed that by the time the average person finally received a diagnosis, they'd been evaluated by various physicians for nine or ten years. Today, the pendulum seems to have swung the other way, and it's become a convenient catchall for a variety of complaints. However, there's no doubt that fibromyalgia is a very real, painful, and sometimes debilitating health condition.

It's estimated that 5 million people in the U.S. have fibromyalgia, and 9 out of 10 sufferers are women.[29] Unfortunately, there is still no specific diagnostic test for this condition. Rather, patients have to meet certain clinical criteria, the most common one being hypersensitivity to pain in very specific areas of the body, including:

- Inside of elbows

- Collarbones

- Inside of knees

- Hips

People also frequently report pain all over their bodies—including in their muscles, ligaments, and tendons—along with a feeling of exhaustion. For these reasons, I'm combining this discussion of fibromyalgia with references to chronic fatigue syndrome and chronic pain as well.

Conventional physicians typically offer some form of pain medication, and perhaps psychotropic drugs like antidepressants. I don't recommend either of these drugs because they do not address the root cause of the problem.

Recent data suggests that central sensitization, in which neurons in your spinal cord become sensitized by inflammation or cell damage, may be involved in the way fibromyalgia sufferers experience pain.[30]

The problem is that fibromyalgia involves a complex array of symptoms including widespread pain and fatigue, and it has multiple causative factors. No one treatment is effective for everyone.

If you have fibromyalgia, chronic fatigue syndrome, or chronic pain, you already know how frustrating it is to manage, and how much confusion you face sorting through all the conflicting nutritional advice about how to eat. The fact is, there's little scientific evidence to support any single eating plan that will work for all sufferers of these conditions.

I believe a high-fat diet will go a long way toward dramatically reducing your symptoms and improving quality of life. It does this by improving your body's ability to produce energy by improving the functioning of your mitochondria.

There is some evidence that people with fibromyalgia experience fewer symptoms if they eliminate one or more of the foods that frequently trigger food allergies or food sensitivities. The most common offenders are corn, wheat, soy, dairy (all of which are highly likely to be contaminated with glyphosate), citrus, and sugar. The top three are pasteurized milk, soy, and gluten (wheat and similar grains). In one study of 17 fibromyalgia patients, nearly half experienced a "significant reduction in pain" after eliminating corn, wheat, dairy, citrus, and sugar.[31]

Science is also beginning to recognize a link between oxidative stress and mitochondrial dysfunction and health issues such as chronic fatigue and fibromyalgia[32]—two conditions that the high-fat diet takes full aim at by bringing the body back into balance.

Although there have been very few studies that look specifically at the effect of a high-fat diet on chronic fatigue syndrome, fibromyalgia, and chronic pain, there was one promising study published in the December 2013 issue of the *Journal of Musculoskeletal Pain*.[33] The diet in this study was expressly nonketogenic (meaning it wasn't designed to promote the production of ketones, either through a high fat content or through regular fasting), but it was low carb. The 33 middle-aged women who followed the diet reported increased energy, less pain, and improved symptom scores on the Fibromyalgia Impact Questionnaire.

If you are dealing with one of these pervasive and difficult to treat conditions, I hope you are empowered by the knowledge that you have the potential to dramatically improve your health and quality of life by changing the nutritional makeup of what you eat, moving away from carbs and toward high-quality fat.

GASTROESOPHAGEAL REFLUX DISEASE (GERD)

The American Gastroenterological Association estimates that 15 million Americans experience daily pain and discomfort from acid reflux, and 60 million suffer from it every month.[34] GERD is responsible for approximately 9 million doctor visits and 5 million hospitalizations a year. In 2014, $5.9 billion was spent just on Nexium[35] (one of the most popular drugs to treat reflux symptoms).

The hallmark symptom of acid reflux is "heartburn"—a burning sensation behind your breastbone that sometimes travels up your throat. In some cases, this pain can be severe enough to be mistaken for a heart attack. Acid reflux occurs when the lower esophageal sphincter relaxes inappropriately, allowing acid from your stomach to flow (reflux) backward into your esophagus.

Mistakenly, acid reflux is thought to be caused by excessive amounts of acid in your stomach, which is why acid-blocking drugs such as Nexium are typically prescribed or recommended. This is a serious medical misconception, as the problem usually results from having *too little* acid in your stomach, and these prescriptions only further reduce acidity. In fact, there are over 16,000 articles in the medical literature showing that suppressing stomach acid does not address the problem. It only temporarily treats the symptoms. To make matters worse, these drugs have side effects, which include magnesium depletion, impaired vitamin B_{12} absorption, and osteoporosis.

The most effective way to treat GERD is to restore balance to the digestive system through diet. The typical Western diet of processed foods and sugars is a surefire way to exacerbate acid reflux as it will upset the bacterial balance in your stomach and intestine, which directly affects your gastric function. MMT is an ideal approach to remedy GERD because it includes plenty of vegetables and other high-quality, unprocessed foods that promote a healthy microbiome and reduce excess weight, which commonly accompanies reflux (37 percent of obese people also have GERD[36]).

Research has shown that adopting a high-fat, low-carb diet can be highly effective in reducing the amount of acid that moves up into the esophagus. A 2006 study published in the journal *Digestive Diseases and Sciences*[37] measured stomach acidity in eight people with GERD before and after they switched to a high-fat, low-carb diet. After just a few days of eating the intervention diet, they experienced significantly fewer symptoms and a reduction in acidity in the lower esophagus. The improvements happened very quickly, which is always motivating when making changes.

Since the high-fat diet has been shown to be an effective weight-loss treatment (see the section on page 282 for more info on this), it can also help treat GERD by removing or greatly reducing a primary contributing factor—obesity. A 2013 study showed that losing weight can significantly reduce GERD symptoms or even resolve them completely. In the study, which was published in the journal *Obesity,* 332 obese adults—both men and women—ate a calorie-restricted diet.[38] After six months, the participants had lost an average of 13 pounds; 65 percent had their GERD completely resolve and 15 percent saw their reflux symptoms partially resolve.

Irritable Bowel Syndrome (IBS)

Irritable bowel syndrome is characterized by digestive symptoms, including abdominal discomfort or pain, bloating, and gas. Some people with IBS experience constipation. Others develop diarrhea. Still others have both simultaneously, or vacillate between the two. IBS is often associated with anxiety and tends to cluster within families.

Since there is no specific test for IBS, it often goes undiagnosed, but experts estimate that up to 11 percent of the global population has symptoms. Approximately twice as many women as men are affected.

Diet plays a major role in IBS, as grains and high-sugar foods feed disease-causing gut bacteria—which can cause gas and gastric upset—and can also trigger serious intestinal inflammation. In my experience, there is usually an underlying emotional stress or anxiety associated with IBS patients, which can go hand in hand with an imbalance in gut bacteria as there is a scientifically recognized connection between gut health and mental health.

Adopting a low-carb diet has been shown to reduce symptoms and improve quality of life in people with IBS. A 2009 study[39] put 13 people with diarrhea-predominant IBS on a four-week diet of less than 20 grams of carbohydrates per day. Participants reported significant reductions in abdominal pain and stool frequency and improvements in stool consistency, and they lost an average of 6.8 pounds. Better yet, 10 of the 13 reported these reductions in symptoms during all four weeks of the trial, meaning the dietary changes yielded fast relief.

More recently, a Japanese study published in the journal *PLoS One* in 2015 looked at the correlation between regular consumption of carbohydrate-rich foods and IBS. This cross-sectional study of 1,082 Japanese adults demonstrated that the consumption of diet staples such as rice, bread, pasta, and buckwheat noodles was associated with a higher prevalence of IBS.[40] A high-fat diet naturally results in consuming fewer carbs, replacing them with plenty of high-fiber vegetables, nuts, and seeds—which in turn feed the good bacteria in your gut. So it stands to reason that these changes will also be helpful in rectifying IBS.

MIGRAINES

More than 37 million Americans suffer from migraines; nearly 5 million of them experience at least one migraine attack per month.[41] In all, an estimated 13 percent of the world's population suffers with migraines to a greater or lesser extent. The condition is more prevalent among women, with about 15 to 18 percent of women worldwide experiencing them, compared to 6 to 7 percent of men.

Despite their prevalence, migraines are still one of the most poorly understood medical disorders out there. Part of the problem has been that the experiences of those suffering from migraines vary greatly. Aside from throbbing, searing pain, which may or may not be one-sided, some experience visual disturbances prior to onset, while others do not. There may also be nausea, vomiting, fever, chills, sweating, and/or sensitivity to light, sound, and smells. The symptoms are also commonly confused with a stroke, as one can lose vision and experience unusual nerve sensations.

Diet does appear to also play a role in migraines: searching the medical literature in PubMed.gov using the search terms "migraine" and "food allergies" will provide you with over 160 different studies.[42] One randomized, double-blind, crossover study published in 2010[43] found that a six-week-long diet that excluded known food allergens produced a statistically significant reduction in the number of migraine attacks and number of headache days.

More recent studies have noted an association between high-fat, low-carb diets and dramatic reductions in migraine attacks. A 2015 study published in the *European Journal of Neurology*[44] assigned 45 women who experienced regular migraines to a ketogenic diet for one month, and then switched them to a standard calorie-restricted diet for another five months. The control group in the study ate a standard calorie-restricted diet for the entire six months. The women eating the high-fat, low-carb diet experienced a significant reduction in the number of attacks, number of days with a headache, and medicine intake during their first month (where the standard, low-calorie dieters didn't). Once they switched to a standard low-calorie diet, their symptoms worsened—although they remained improved compared to baseline. The group who didn't start with the ketogenic diet did see a reduction in the number of days with a headache—but not until month three, and they did not see a reduction in attack frequency until month six. Which would you prefer—noticeable relief within one month, or waiting three to six months?

A fascinating 2013 Italian study published in *Functional Neurology*[45] reported a case where 47-year-old twin sisters adopted a low-carb, high-fat weight-loss diet. After three days on the diet, their frequent migraines also "unexpectedly vanished." The sisters ate a ketogenic diet for four weeks and then transitioned to a low-calorie, non-ketogenic diet for two months before starting the ketogenic diet cycle again.

Before starting the diet, the sisters suffered from five to seven migraine attacks a month. They experienced no headaches while on the high-fat, four-week cycle. Their migraines did recur during the two-month, nonketogenic intervals, although with reduced frequency, duration, and intensity. The researchers theorized that the diet reduced inflammation and oxidative stress in the neurons of the patients and enhanced mitochondrial genetics, which in turn resulted in a dramatic reduction in migraine attacks.

MULTIPLE SCLEROSIS

Multiple sclerosis (MS) is a chronic, degenerative disease involving the brain and spinal column caused by demyelination of the nerves. Myelin is the insulating, waxy substance that surrounds the nerves in your central nervous system. When the myelin is damaged by self-destructive processes, the function of those nerves deteriorates over time, resulting in a number of symptoms, including:

- Muscle weakness
- Sensory disturbances
- Cognition and memory problems
- Imbalance, or loss of coordination
- Astigmatism and vision loss
- Tremors

MS may progress steadily or present as acute attacks followed by a temporary remission of symptoms. Previous studies have shown that vitamin D can positively impact MS by altering chemicals called cytokines, which modulate your immune system. Therefore, one of the best strategies you can implement for your health in general is also one of the best preventive strategies against autoimmune diseases like MS: getting enough regular sun exposure so your body can produce optimal amounts of vitamin D.

Studies have found that higher blood levels of vitamin D help protect against the development of MS, so if you don't have access to regular sensible sun exposure, or a safe tanning bed, you may want to seriously consider oral supplementation with vitamin D_3.

One such study, published in 2004, found that women who took vitamin D–containing multivitamin supplements were 40 percent less likely to develop MS than women who did not supplement.[46] Keep in mind that this study was based on *far* lower dosages of vitamin D than what we now know are needed, so if you optimize your levels, you're likely to reduce your risk by far more than 40 percent.

While research on high-fat diets and multiple sclerosis is still emerging, it is promising. One 2012 animal study looked at the effects of a ketogenic diet on memory impairment and neuroinflammation—two hallmarks of MS. The mice fed the high-fat diet had fewer markers of inflammation and lower levels of reactive oxygen species (which, as you have learned, damage cells through oxidation). They also improved their performance on tests of spatial learning, memory, and motor ability.[47]

There is a growing body of evidence suggesting that mitochondrial dysfunction is at the root of neurodegenerative diseases, including MS,[48] which suggests that a diet that improves mitochondrial health, as MMT does, will also help manage and treat MS symptoms.[49]

Nonalcoholic Fatty Liver Disease

Nonalcoholic fatty liver disease (NAFLD) is defined as an excessive accumulation of fats in your liver—more than 5 to 10 percent of the total weight of the liver—in the absence of significant alcohol consumption. While it's normal for your liver to contain some fat, when levels get too high your liver can no longer regulate your blood sugar, which leads to a cascade of serious health problems. If left untreated, NAFLD can cause your liver to swell or even contribute to liver cancer or liver failure.

Interestingly, the fat that gets stored in your liver in the form of triglycerides does *not* come from eating fatty foods. It comes from eating a diet rich in carbohydrates. This is why ducks and geese are force-fed corn to make foie gras (French for "fatty liver"). The sugar-rich American diet is a likely contributor to the current epidemic of NAFLD—25 percent of adults[50] and 10 percent of children in America have this disease,[51] which was almost unheard of in not-so-distant past. Fructose, which is the sugar found in most processed foods (often in the form of high-fructose corn syrup) can *only* be metabolized by your liver.

Nearly all fructose gets shuttled to your liver. And if you eat a typical Western-style diet, you consume high amounts of it. The overload of fructose ends up taxing and damaging your liver in the same way alcohol and other toxins do. You don't even need to be wildly overdoing it on the fructose front to be putting your liver at risk: a 2015 study from Tufts University revealed that those who consumed at least one sugary drink daily had a higher risk of liver damage and NAFLD.[52]

The good news is that dramatically reducing the number of carbs you eat has been shown to have powerful benefits in NAFLD. A 2011 study published in the *American Journal of Clinical Nutrition*[53] assigned two groups of patients with NAFLD to either a low-calorie or a low-carbohydrate diet for two weeks. At the end of the intervention, both groups had lost weight and lowered their triglycerides, but the low-carb group had a significantly greater reduction in liver fat. *In only two weeks.*

A 2011 Spanish pilot study published in the *Journal of Medicinal Food* placed 14 men with NAFLD on a Spanish ketogenic Mediterranean diet for 12 weeks. After those three months, 100 percent of the men had normal triglyceride and HDL cholesterol levels, 21 percent had completely resolved their NAFLD, and 92 percent had an overall reduction in the fat stored in their liver.[54]

An earlier study from 2007[55] found similar results, when five men with NAFLD were placed on a low-carb, ketogenic diet and followed for six months. Of the four who stuck with the eating regimen, their follow-up biopsies revealed a significant reduction in the percentage of fat in their livers. They also had improvements in the scarring—known as fibrosis—that can accompany NAFLD, and they lost a mean of 28 pounds.

OBESITY

Two out of three Americans are now either overweight or obese. As a 2014 article in the *New York Times* noted,[56] the weight of the average American increased by 24 pounds in the four decades between the 1960s and 2002.

But it's not just a problem of size: in the U.S., just eight obesity-related diseases—including type 2 diabetes, hypertension, heart disease, nonalcoholic fatty liver disease, dementia, and cancer—account for 75 percent of all health care costs!

Keep in mind, however, that while obesity is associated with these diseases, it is not their *cause*. Obesity is a *marker*. The underlying problem, linking obesity with all of these health issues, is *metabolic dysfunction*. And the primary driver of metabolic dysfunction is insulin resistance, which in turn is typically caused by excessive consumption of carbohydrates. This means that your weight gain could be a sign that your overall health may be in jeopardy. Contrary to popular belief, obesity is not simply the result of eating too many calories and not exercising enough.

As Dr. Malcolm Kendrick, author of *Doctoring Data: How to Sort Out Medical Advice from Medical Nonsense*, notes, much of the medical advice we take as gospel is simply *made up*. There's no support and no science for it, and the "calorie theory" appears to fall into this category.

While there's science to show the actual number of calories in a pound of fat, it's a major flaw in logic to say that all you have to do to *lose* that pound of fat is to create an equal caloric deficit. (Zoë Harcombe's book, *The Obesity Epidemic: What Caused It? How*

Can We Stop It? is the most comprehensive document on this topic that I've come across, and exposes this flaw in the science. If you'd like to dive deeper into this topic, her book and Dr. Kendrick's are great places to start.)

While I know it can be difficult to let go of the idea that what you need to do to lose weight is eat fewer calories and exercise more, the good news in all this is that you *can* shed excess pounds by choosing *different* sources for your calories. When you shift your diet away from a steady stream of nonfiber carbs, and integrate regular periods of feasting and fasting, you allow your body to recalibrate its sensitivity to insulin. And when you replace those nonfiber carbs with high-quality fats, you empower your body to start burning its fat stores for fuel, which helps the weight come off. Better yet, the fats help you feel full and satisfied, making adherence to this diet much easier to maintain than low-calorie or low-fat diets.

TRAUMATIC BRAIN INJURY

According to the CDC, some 1.7 million traumatic brain injuries occur in the U.S. each year, many of them resulting from sports injuries or automobile accidents.

Once a person with a traumatic brain injury is stabilized, there is no standard treatment to help their brain recover; most physicians, instead, adopt a "wait and see" approach to determine if the person will regain neurological function.

Sixty percent of your brain is made up of fat. DHA alone makes up about 15 percent to 20 percent of your brain's cerebral cortex. It's found in high levels in your neurons—the cells of your central nervous system—where it provides structural support.

Because your brain is literally built from fats, it makes sense that high doses of the most beneficial ones following injury could support your brain's natural healing process. In particular, science has evaluated the effect of two specific fat-related substances:

- Omega-3 fats
- Ketones, which your body produces when you consume a high-fat, low-net-carb, moderate-protein diet

How might omega-3 fats help the brain heal from a traumatic injury? They are known to:

- Inhibit cell death[57]
- Help reconnect damaged neurons[58]
- Activate genes that help cope with brain damage while turning off those that promote brain inflammation[59]

There have been documented cases of patients making remarkable recoveries from brain injuries after supplementing with omega-3 fats.[60, 61] Unfortunately, this is still considered an "unorthodox" treatment for traumatic brain injury, and is not routinely ordered as a standard of care, primarily because large-scale human trials have yet to be conducted—and are not likely to be conducted since omega-3 fats are widely available over the counter and thus are not easily patentable by pharmaceutical companies. But despite the pharmaceutical industry's indifference, here's what we do know:

- Brain injuries impair glucose metabolism in the brain,[62] while eating a high-fat, low-net-carb diet produces ketones, which the brain can use as an alternate fuel to glucose.

- Brain injuries result in neuroinflammation (inflammation in your nervous system);[63] ketones and a high-fat diet are anti-inflammatory.

- Over time, brain injuries can result in epileptic seizures,[64] and ketogenic diets have been shown to dramatically reduce the frequency of seizures.

- Rats fed a ketogenic diet after brain injury experienced a reduction in contusion volume (injured area).[65]

- They also experienced decreased swelling and cell death.[66]

If restoring brain health is a challenge you or a loved one is facing after a traumatic injury, the high-fat diet can provide the vital building blocks the brain needs to repair itself.

Type 2 Diabetes

In the U.S., 115 million people—or nearly one in three[67]—has some form of diabetes or pre-diabetes. Nearly 28 percent of people with diabetes do not know they have it,[68] which increases the odds of developing potentially deadly complications.

The most recent data, released in 2014, reveals that between 2001 and 2009, incidence of type 2 diabetes among children aged 10 to 19 rose by 30 percent![69] I use an exclamation point because type 2 diabetes had always been considered an adult disease. Now the epidemic is even affecting our children.

Statistics such as these point to two very important facts. First, they tell us that diabetes cannot be primarily caused by genetics, and second, they scream that something we're doing, consistently and en masse, is horribly wrong and we need to address the problem head-on.

Conventional medicine has type 2 diabetes pegged as a problem with blood sugar control but this is a misperception. The reality is that diabetes is a disease rooted in *insulin resistance*, which is typically caused by a diet that is too high in sugars and carbs. When you have insulin resistance, you have plenty of insulin circulating in your blood, to the point that insulin receptors become desensitized to it.

Even science is starting to understand that insulin is not the way to treat type 2 diabetes:

A study published in the June 30, 2014, issue of *JAMA Internal Medicine*[70] concluded that insulin therapy in type 2 diabetic patients may indeed do more harm than good. And yet, conventional medicine continues to prescribe insulin to treat high blood glucose levels. On top of that, conventionally trained doctors pass along this seriously flawed nutritional information to diabetic patients, allowing the disease to expand to epidemic proportions.

While much conventional advice centers on insulin, *leptin* is another hormone that plays an integral role in the development of type 2 diabetes. Leptin is produced primarily in your fat cells, and one of its primary roles is regulating your appetite and body weight. Leptin tells your brain when to eat, how much to eat, and most importantly, when to stop eating. Leptin also tells your brain what to do with the available energy.

When your blood sugar is elevated, *insulin* is released to direct the extra energy into storage, the majority of which is stored as *fat*, and *leptin* is produced in these fat cells. The more fat you have, the more leptin is produced. This is why I typically talk about insulin *and* leptin resistance, as they work in tandem. Moreover, *leptin is largely responsible for the accuracy of insulin signaling and whether or not you become insulin resistant.* If you're insulin resistant, most likely you're leptin resistant as well, especially if you're overweight or obese. Just as with insulin, the only known way to reestablish proper leptin signaling is through proper diet.

High consumption of carbohydrates, especially fructose, is the prime culprit in both insulin and leptin resistance, which means that changing your diet has enormous potential to correct both of these major triggers of type 2 diabetes.

A high-fat diet appears to be particularly promising for treating diabetes.

Dr. Charles Mobbs, an animal researcher at the Icahn School of Medicine at Mount Sinai in New York City, published a study in the journal *PLoS One* in 2011[71] reporting he found that mice with type 1 diabetes and type 2 diabetes with early-stage kidney disease experienced a complete reversal of their kidney disease after eight weeks on a high-fat, ketogenic diet (87 percent fat). A similar reversal in humans could mean avoiding dialysis.

A 2015 critical review of previous studies published in the journal *Nutrition*[72] amassed evidence of the ways a low-carb, high-fat diet improves diabetes. Of these, the most crucial were twofold:

First, limiting carbohydrates is a proven way of significantly lowering blood sugar, even more effective than simply limiting calories. And second, following a high-fat diet has been shown multiple times to result in less need for medication in type 2 diabetics. Of course, a high-fat diet is also known to be highly effective in reducing excess weight, which is a known trigger for type 2 diabetes.

Despite the flawed advice from the American Diabetes Association, which is still recommending that diabetics eat ¾ to 1 cup of high net carbs *at every meal*,[73] your best bet in managing—or even reversing—your type 2 diabetes is to adopt a low-carb, high-fat diet.

APPENDIX B

A Guide to Nuts and Seeds

Cacao Powder, Nibs, and Butter

Most of us love chocolate but few know that it is derived from the fruit of an odd-sounding tree called cacao.

Cacao can be purchased as nibs, powder, or butter. Raw cacao powder has nearly four times the antioxidants of regular dark chocolate, making it one of the most concentrated sources of antioxidants available. In addition, it contains protein, calcium, carotene, thiamine, riboflavin, magnesium, sulfur, and more than 380 phytochemicals.

One of the best ways to consume cacao powder is to buy raw cacao nibs and then grind them into powder in a small coffee grinder just before using. Or you can purchase raw cacao butter, which is far less bitter and easier to tolerate, although it has fewer antioxidants than nibs or powder. Ideally both should be organic and Fair Trade.

How to eat it: Cacao powder and butter both taste great added to a smoothie with a small amount of a natural sweetener—you can use either or both. I find that stevia works best to convert the cacao powder into a delicious treat, and I have three small smoothies a day with it. It contains no polyunsaturated fat at all, so you don't have to worry about cacao powder nudging your omega-6 fat intake too high, as you do with most all other nuts and seeds on this list. Cacao butter can also be used wherever you would use butter.

BLACK SESAME

You may have eaten sesame seeds on a bagel, but black sesame seeds are a totally different food. Unlike white sesame seeds, black sesame seeds are unhulled, giving them a more complex flavor and delivering a wallop of additional nutritional benefits.

The Traditional Chinese Medicine classic text the *Compendium of Materia Medica*, written during the Ming Dynasty, says, "Taking black sesame seeds can heal all the chronic illness after 100 days, improve skin tone on body and face after 1 year, reverse gray hair after 2 years, and regrow teeth after 3 years."

Black sesame seeds have more calcium per gram than any other food and are excellent sources of magnesium, copper, and zinc, making them one of nature's multivitamins. They are also rich in lignans, a type of plant compound rich in polyphenols and insoluble fiber. Once ingested, lignans are converted into weak forms of estrogen that help regulate hormone balance in the body, and can potentially help reduce the risk of hormone-associated cancers (breast, uterine, ovarian, and prostate). There is research suggesting that postmenopausal women who have a high intake of dietary lignans have a 17 percent lower risk of breast cancer compared to those with a low intake.[1]

How to eat: Toss one ounce of seeds in a stir-fry of low-carb vegetables, sprinkle a small handful over a salad, or even eat them straight, making sure to chew them well and not just swallow them. Or you can add a tablespoon to a smoothie along with some of the other seeds on the list.

Flax Seeds

Humans have long grown flax and used it to make linen fabric, but its usefulness is just as applicable to the inside of the body as it is to the outside. Flax seeds' beneficial properties fall into three major categories:

- Flax seeds are a rich source of omega-3 fats, in the form of the anti-inflammatory alpha-linolenic acid.

- Lignans, as discussed in the black sesame seed entry, are insoluble fibers and polyphenols that your body converts into weak forms of phytoestrogens. Flax seeds provide substantially more lignans than black sesame seeds—approximately 10 times the amount.

- Flax seeds are an excellent source of fiber, both soluble and insoluble.

How to eat flax seeds: Whole flax seeds can be freshly ground (in an inexpensive coffee or spice grinder) just prior to eating. Even better would to soak them overnight and add them to the blender when you make your smoothie. You can use about a tablespoon in your smoothie, or sprinkle freshly ground flax meal into smoothies, vegetable juices, or soup; add them to eggs or guacamole (their subtle, nutty flavor won't overpower); and use them in place of bread crumbs in meatballs or crab cakes.

An important caution here is to avoid using pre-ground flax seeds or even worse, flax seed oil (which is advocated on the Budwig Cancer Protocol). Please understand that nearly all flax seed oil is seriously oxidized and should be discarded. It is easily replaced with the equivalent amount of soaked flax seeds.

Remember: one of the most important principles of MMT is to use the highest-quality and freshest ingredients possible, which will maximize the health benefits of using this approach.

CHIA SEEDS

Chia seeds were a prized food to the ancient Aztecs and Mayans. *Chia* is the ancient Mayan word for strength, and the tiny seeds were valued for their energy-boosting properties.

Chia seeds are a quick and easy-to-use source of protein, healthy omega-3 fats, dietary fiber, minerals, vitamins, and antioxidants, all rolled into one tiny package. Although they have similar health benefits to flax seeds, chia seeds don't have to be ground prior to consumption, and they don't go rancid as quickly either. In fact, chia seeds are said to last up to two years with no refrigeration, courtesy of the high levels of antioxidants they contain.

Perhaps their greatest benefit is their high amount of fiber: just one tablespoon of chia seeds contains about 5 grams of fiber.

How to eat: When chia seeds are soaked in water or coconut milk overnight, they take on a tapioca-like texture; add some cinnamon and/or raw cacao powder and a bit of stevia for a pudding-like treat that can be eaten any time. You can also sprinkle chia seeds over smoothies or soups, but they do absorb water and become gelatinous, so if it's crunch you're after, sprinkle them on just before eating. Or sprout your chia seeds (yes, just like with a Chia Pet) and eat these nutritional superstars in salads or on their own.

Caution: If you have a history of difficulty swallowing, or are giving chia seeds to children, take care not to eat a handful of them and then immediately drink water, as they can quickly form a gel-like ball that can partially block the esophagus, requiring medical treatment to remove.

BLACK CUMIN

Black cumin, also known as black seed, black caraway, onion seed, and Roman coriander, has a long history of use in traditional systems of medicine, including Ayurveda. The prophet Mohammed even described this humble black seed as a cure for every disease but death itself. It is important to understand that black cumin seeds are not the same as the cumin spice. They are not as easy to find in grocery stores as some of the other seeds but can easily be found online.

More than 650 peer-reviewed studies have looked into the potential health benefits of "black seed" and have found it to have antimicrobial, liver-protective, immune-supporting, analgesic, antispasmodic, and antioxidant properties.[2]

Black cumin may also have anti-obesity effects, including reductions in body weight and waist and hip circumference.[3]

How to eat it: With a warm, slightly bitter flavor that tastes something like a blend of thyme, oregano, and nutmeg, black cumin is a palatable addition to your diet. You can add the seeds to casseroles, stir-fries, and salad dressings (try them mixed with lemon, cilantro, and tahini); sprinkle them on salads; or even add them to your coffee or tea. You can also make black cumin tea by pouring hot water over the seeds (about one tablespoon) and letting it steep for 10 minutes. I add about one tablespoon (or 11 grams) of black cumin seeds to my breakfast smoothie every morning.

SUNFLOWER SEEDS

Though made famous in paintings by Van Gogh, and for populating entire fields in the south of France, sunflowers are actually North America natives. They were cultivated by Native Americans as early as 3000 B.C. and used as food and as a source of oil, and even ground into flour.

Sunflower seeds are rich in vitamin E, copper, B vitamins, manganese, selenium, phosphorus, and magnesium. Vitamin E is a potent antioxidant that protects cell membranes and cholesterol from free radical damage, giving it powerful anti-inflammatory properties.

How to eat them: I firmly believe that the best way to consume sunflower seeds is to sprout them. Spouts in general are a powerful delivery system of raw, living nutrients, and sunflower sprouts are the most nutrient dense of all sprouts—about 30 times more nutrient dense than most vegetables. Seek to include a few ounces regularly in your salads. They are expensive to purchase (about $30 per pound) but cost well under $1 per pound if you grow them yourself. (Go to mercola.com and search for "sprouting seeds" for more information on how to do this.)

Sunflower seeds are also great on their own as a snack. Mix them into high-fat, grass-fed burgers, add them to a grain-free granola, sprinkle them over a salad for a refreshing texture addition, or use a high-powered blender to grind them into sunflower butter. As sunflower seeds have a high omega-6 oil content, they spoil easily; keep them in the refrigerator or freezer if possible, and definitely away from light.

Pumpkin Seeds

If you're in the mood for a crunchy snack that doubles as a phenomenal health food, look no further than pumpkin seeds. With a wide variety of nutrients ranging from magnesium and manganese to copper, protein, and zinc, pumpkin seeds are nutritional powerhouses wrapped up in a very small package.

Magnesium participates in the creation of ATP, the synthesis of RNA and DNA, the pumping of your heart, proper bone and tooth formation, relaxation of your blood vessels, and proper bowel function. Magnesium has been shown to benefit your blood pressure and help prevent sudden cardiac arrest, heart attack, and stroke. Yet an estimated 80 percent of Americans are deficient in this important mineral.

Like sunflower seeds, pumpkin seeds also contain high levels of phytosterols and free radical–scavenging antioxidants. They are also high in fiber.

Pumpkin seeds are a rich source of zinc (one ounce contains more than 2 mg of this beneficial mineral). Zinc is important to your body in many ways, including immunity, cell growth and division, sleep, and mood. Zinc is also important for prostate health (where it is found in the highest concentrations in the body).[4]

How to eat them: Raw pumpkin seeds are great on their own. They are also a good addition to grain-free granola, salads, and soups, or freshly ground and added to your smoothie.

PSYLLIUM SEED HUSKS

If you're looking for a healthy way to supplement your fiber intake—which is an important part of Mitochondrial Metabolic Therapy—organic, whole-husk psyllium is a simple, cost-effective way to do it. Psyllium is a high-fiber food source that is actually the ground husks of the seeds of the *Plantago ovata* plant. It contains both soluble and insoluble fiber, which have a long list of important attributes that contribute to physical health, as I covered in Chapter 5.

Taking psyllium three times a day could add as much as 18 grams of dietary fiber (soluble and insoluble) to your diet, which brings you quite close to the recommended minimum of 50 grams per 1,000 calories consumed—although please understand that using psyllium is not a replacement for eating plenty of fiber in the form of vegetables. This level of psyllium would have to be worked up to gradually and may not be necessary for everyone.

Caution: If you suspect that you have a bowel obstruction or have a history of bowel adhesions, only take psyllium under appropriate medical supervision.

How to eat it: Psyllium is perfect for adding to smoothies, as it blends well and changes their texture, making them thicker. You can also mix one heaping tablespoon in a glass of water three times a day, and follow it with another glass of water to help the fiber pass through your system. Please keep in mind that psyllium is a heavily sprayed crop, which means many common sources are contaminated with pesticides, herbicides, and fertilizers. For this reason, be sure to *only* use organic psyllium husk, and make sure it's 100 percent pure: many supplement brands use synthetic or semi-synthetic active ingredients that do *not* contain psyllium, such as methylcellulose and calcium polycarbophil. I also recommend choosing a psyllium powder that does not contain additives or sweeteners, as these tend to have a detrimental effect on your microbiome. Sugar in particular feeds potentially pathogenic microorganisms, which is the opposite of what you're trying to achieve. It also adds to your overall carb count, and this is counterproductive to the aims of MMT. Also be wary of artificial sweeteners. Research is slowly building the case that these foreign foods can lower the number of beneficial bacteria, resulting in a negative impact on your microbiome.

MACADAMIA NUTS

When you think of macadamia nuts, Hawaii might come to mind, but this nut is actually native to the continent Down Under, which explains why the fruit is also known as the Australian or Queensland nut. These are some of the most sought-after nuts in the world, so expect to pay more.

Macadamia nuts have the highest fat and lowest protein and carb content of any nut, and they also happen to be one of my favorites. Raw macadamia nuts also contain high amounts of vitamin B_1, magnesium, and manganese. Just one serving of macadamia nuts nets 58 percent of what you need in manganese, and 23 percent of the recommended daily value of thiamine.

About 80 percent of the fats in macadamia nuts are monounsaturated, and most of those fats are the omega-9 fat, oleic acid. This is the same fat that is also present in olive oil, so they provide many of the same benefits as olive oil. They are typically less oxidized than olive oil because the fat is intact, not extracted (if you consume them, as recommended, as a fresh, raw nut).

If you have pets, it's important to note that macadamia nuts are toxic to dogs and can cause weakness, vomiting, loss of coordination, tremors, and hyperthermia.

How to eat: These tasty nuts are a perfect snack eaten on their own. You can grind them into nut butter, chop them finely and use them to "bread" meat or fish, chop them more coarsely and add them to a salad, or mix them into soups for a little crunch. Keep your consumption to 60 grams or less a day.

Pecans

The pecan tree traces its origins to North America. Throughout millennia, pecans were an important staple in the Native American food supply. And Native Americans were instrumental in teaching the early colonists how to harvest, utilize, and store pecans as an essential source of nourishment to tap into during harsh winters.

Pecans contain more than 19 vitamins and minerals, and research has suggested that they lower LDL cholesterol and promote healthy arterial function.[5] Pecans are a close second to macadamia nuts on the fat and protein scale, and they also contain anti-inflammatory magnesium, heart-healthy oleic acid, phenolic antioxidants, and immune-boosting manganese.

Pecans are in the top 15 foods identified by the USDA as high in antioxidant activity. Pecans are also chock-full of minerals including manganese, which is not easily obtained from your diet.

How to eat them: Raw pecans are delicious eaten on their own, or chopped and combined with coconut oil, ground cacao nibs, cinnamon, and a little bit of stevia for a sweet treat. For a truly delicious savory snack, toss raw pecans in butter and sprinkle them with sea salt and then roast them using low heat.

Brazil Nuts

Brazil nuts are a nutrient-dense and delicious type of nut that comes from a tree in South America that bears the same name.

Brazil nuts are most notable as an excellent source of selenium, an essential mineral that may be beneficial in preventing cancer and other chronic diseases and as an antagonist to mercury. They also have a high-fat and low-protein content, following closely behind macadamias and pecans. And they are rich in zinc; this is important given that so many Americans are deficient in this mineral.

There is a long and impressive list of health benefits associated with Brazil nuts, including their ability to help stimulate growth and repair, improve the digestive process, boost heart health, balance hormone function, improve the immune system, lower risk of cancer, boost male fertility, help with weight loss, aid in skin health, and reduce the signs of aging.

Brazil nuts also contain the amino acid l-arginine, which offers multiple vascular benefits to people with heart disease or to those who have increased risk for heart disease due to multiple cardiac risk factors.

Despite their many health benefits, eating more than a few per day has downsides. For one, you can easily exceed your ideal intake of selenium and that can have a negative impact on your health. Also, due to their extensive root systems, Brazil nuts contain small amounts of radium.[6]

How to eat them: Brazil nuts are great eaten whole. It is important to eat shelled Brazil nuts quickly, as the high fat content makes these nut varieties go bad quite quickly. Like the other nuts listed in this section, they can also be chopped and sprinkled over other foods included in the MMT protocol.

Almonds

Almonds are technically not a nut; they're a seed. The almond tree is in the same family as peach, apricot, and cherry trees, and like those cousins, almond trees bear fruit that have a stony seed, or pit. The almond is that pit.

Almonds contain l-arginine and are also good sources of potassium, a mineral that helps normalize blood pressure.

Do be careful not to overeat almonds, however, as they are high in protein: four almonds contain nearly 1 gram. They are also relatively high in omega-6 fats, about 30 percent, so too many will distort your healthy omega-6-to-omega-3 ratio. The have about 60 percent saturated fats and only 10 percent monounsaturated fat.

It can be difficult to find truly raw almonds in the U.S. because almonds sold in North America can still be labeled "raw" even though they've been subjected to one of the following pasteurization methods:

- Oil roasting, dry roasting, or blanching
- Steam processing
- Propylene oxide (PPO) treatment (PPO is a highly toxic flammable chemical compound, once used as a racing fuel before it was prohibited for safety reasons)

It *is* possible to purchase raw almonds in the U.S., but it has to be done through vendors who sell small quantities of genuinely raw almonds and have obtained a waiver from the pasteurization requirement. The key is to find a company with this waiver.

If you do choose to consume almonds, you may want to soak them first. This will help rid them of the phytic acid and enzyme inhibitors they naturally contain. Enzyme inhibitors in nuts (and seeds) help protect the nut as it grows, decreasing enzyme activity and preventing premature sprouting. But in your body, these enzymes can interfere with the function of your own digestive and metabolic enzymes. To make soaked nuts more palatable, you can use a dehydrator to improve the texture.

How to eat: Of course, you can simply snack on almonds. You can also grind them into almond butter using a high-powered blender and spread it on celery, or mix it into smoothies with ground cacao nibs for a nutty, chocolatey treat. Store almonds in a dark cabinet, the refrigerator, or the freezer to preserve freshness and prevent rancidity.

I personally don't eat any almonds because I want to keep my omega-6 content low, but they can be used in a limited amount. It's probably best to limit them, like seeds, to about 15 grams per day.

Nutrient Levels of MMT-Friendly Nuts and Seeds

Note: Values are based on volume measurement of one level tablespoon, which makes measuring easy. There is a wide range of weights, from 4 grams with psyllium to 11 grams with cacao nibs.

Seed/Nut	Fat	Protein	F/P	Carbs	Fiber	C/F
Cacao Nibs	4.7	1.6	2.9	3.9	3.5	1.1
Black Sesame	5.2	1.8	2.9	2.8	1.5	1.9
Flax	4.2	1.8	2.3	2.9	2.7	1.1
Chia	2.8	1.5	1.9	3.8	3.1	1.2
Hemp	2.1	1.5	1.4	1.7	1.7	1.0
Black Cumin	1.5	1.2	1.3	3.0	0.8	3.8
Sunflower	2.1	1.8	1.2	2.7	0.8	3.4
Pumpkin	1.7	1.7	1.0	4.8	1.7	2.8
Psyllium	0	0	0	4.0	4.0	1.0
Macadamia	7.6	0.8	9.5	1.4	0.9	1.6
Pecan	7.2	1.4	5.1	1.4	1.0	1.4
Brazil	6.6	1.4	4.7	1.2	0.8	1.5
Almond	4.0	1.7	2.4	1.7	1.9	0.9

ENDNOTES

Introduction

1   K. M. Adams, W. S. Butsch, and M. Kohlmeier, "The State of Nutrition Education at US Medical Schools," *Journal of Biomedical Education*, vol. 2015 (January 2015), Article ID 357627, 7 pages. DOI:10.1155/2015/357627.

2   "Cancer Facts & Figures 2016," American Cancer Society, Atlanta, Georgia, 2016, http://www.cancer.org/acs/groups/content/@research/documents/document/acspc-047079.pdf, accessed 12/2/16.

3   "Global Cancer Facts & Figures, 3rd Edition," American Cancer Society, Atlanta, Georgia, 2015, http://www.cancer.org/acs/groups/content/@research/documents/document/acspc-044738.pdf, accessed 12/2/16.

4   N. Howlader et al. (eds.), "SEER Cancer Statistics Review, 1975–2013," National Cancer Institute, Bethesda, MD, April 2016, http://seer.cancer.gov/csr/1975_2013/, accessed 12/2/16.

5   M. Harper, "David Graham on the Vioxx Verdict," Forbes.com, August 19, 2005, http://www.forbes.com/2005/08/19/merck-vioxx-graham_cx_mh_0819graham.html, accessed 12/2/16.

Chapter 1

1   N. Lane, *Power, Sex, Suicide: Mitochondria and the Meaning of Life* (New York: Oxford University Press, 2006), 3.

2   Ibid.

3   Ibid, location 5926.

4   "Our Best Days Are Yours," Kellogg's, https://www.kelloggs.com/en_US/who-we-are/our-history.html, accessed 12/2/16.

5   L. B. Wrenn, *Cinderella of the New South* (Knoxville, TN: University of Tennessee Press, 1995), 84.

6   T. G. Graham and D. Ramsey, *The Happiness Diet* (New York: Rodale Books, 2012), 25.

7   F. G. Mather, "Waste Products: Cotton-Seed Oil," *Popular Science Monthly*, May 1894, 104.

8   Graham and Ramsey, *The Happiness Diet*.

9   "Our Heritage," Crisco, http://www.crisco.com/about_crisco/history.aspx, accessed 12/2/16.

10   S. Gokhale, "Marketing Crisco," Weston A. Price Foundation, June 25, 2013, http://www.westonaprice.org/health-topics/marketing-crisco/, accessed 12/2/16.

11   Graham and Ramsey, *The Happiness Diet.*

12   T. L. Blasbalg et al., "Changes in Consumption of Omega-3 and Omega-6 Fatty Acids in the United States During the 20th Century," *American Journal of Clinical Nutrition*, 93, no. 5 (May 2011): 950–62: DOI: 10.3945/ajcn.110.006643. Epub 2011 Mar 2.

13   S. F. Halabi, *Food and Drug Regulation in an Era of Globalized Markets* (Cambridge, MA: Academic Press, 2015), 148.

14   T. Neltner, M. Maffini, "Generally Recognized as Secret: Chemicals Added to Food in the United States," National Resources Defense Council, April 2014, https://www.nrdc.org/sites/default/files/safety-loophole-for-chemicals-in-food -report.pdf, accessed 12/2/16.

15   R. J. de Souza et al., "Intake of Saturated and Trans Unsaturated Fatty Acids and Risk of All Cause Mortality, Cardiovascular Disease, and Type 2 Diabetes: Systematic Review and Meta-analysis of Observational Studies," *BMJ* (2015): 351, DOI: 10.1136/bmj.h3978.

16   V. T. Samuel, K. F. Petersen, and G. I. Shulman, "Lipid-induced Insulin Resistance: Unraveling the Mechanism," *Lancet*, 375, (2010): 2267–77, DOI: 10.1016/S0140-6736(10)60408-4.

17   K. Kavanagh et al., "Trans Fat Diet Induces Abdominal Obesity and Changes in Insulin Sensitivity in Monkeys," *Obesity*, 15, no. 7 (July 2007): 1675–84, DOI: 10.1038/oby.2007.200.

18   M. C. Morris et al., "Dietary fats and the risk of incident Alzheimer's disease," *Archives of Neurology*, 60, no. 2 (2003):194–200, DOI: 10.1001 /archneur.60.2.194.

19   C. M. Benbrook, "Impacts of Genetically Engineered Crops on Pesticide Use in the U.S.—the First Sixteen Years," *Environmental Sciences Europe*, 24, no. 1 (2012): 24, DOI: 10.1186/2190-4715-24-24.

20   N. Defarge et al., "Co-Formulants in Glyphosate-Based Herbicides Disrupt Aromatase Activity in Human Cells below Toxic Levels," *International Journal of Environmental Research and Public Health*, 13, no. 3 (2016): 264, DOI: 10.3390 /ijerph13030264.

21   A. Keys, "Mediterranean Diet and Public Health: Personal Reflections," *American Journal of Clinical Nutrition,* 61, no. 6 supplement (1995): 1321S–1323S.

22   A. Keys, "Atherosclerosis: A Problem in Newer Public Health," *Journal of Mt. Sinai Hospital*, New York, 20, no. 2 (July–August 1953): 134.

23   N. Teichholz, *The Big Fat Surprise* (New York: Simon & Schuster, 2014), 32–33.

24   Central Committee for Medical and Community Program of the American Heart Association, "Dietary Fat and Its Relation to Heart Attacks and Strokes," *Circulation* 23 (1961): 133–36. http://circ.ahajournals.org/content /circulationaha/23/1/133.full.pdf, accessed 12/2/16.

25   H. M. Marvin, *1924–1964: The 40 Year War on Heart Disease* (New York: American Heart Association, 1964).

26   A. Keys, "Coronary Heart Disease in Seven Countries," *Circulation*, 41, no. 1 (1970): 1186–95.

27   Dietary Guidelines Advisory Committee, "History of the Dietary Guidelines for Americans," *Nutrition and Health: Dietary Guidelines for Americans, 2005*, U.S. Department of Health and Human Services, https://health.gov /dietaryguidelines/dga2005/report/html/G5_History.htm, accessed 12/2/16.

28   Z. Harcombe et al., "Evidence from Randomised Controlled Trials Did Not Support the Introduction of Dietary Fat Guidelines in 1977 and 1983: A Systematic Review and Meta-analysis," *Open Heart*, 2, no. 1 (2015): DOI: 10.1136/openhrt-2014-000196.

29   U.S. Department of Health and Human Services and U.S. Department of Agriculture, "Key Recommendations: Components of Healthy Eating Patterns," 2015–2020 *Dietary Guidelines for Americans, 8th Edition* (December 2015): 15, https://health.gov/dietaryguidelines/2015/guidelines/chapter-1/key -recommendations/#footnote-4, accessed 12/2/16.

30   Centers for Disease Control and Prevention, Division of Diabetes Translation, "Long-term Trends in Diabetes," (2016). https://www.cdc.gov/diabetes /statistics/slides/long_term_trends.pdf.

31   C. D. Fryar, M. Carroll, and C. Ogden, Division of Health and Nutrition Examination Surveys, "Prevalence of Overweight, Obesity, and Extreme Obesity Among Adults Aged 20 and Over: United States, 1960–1962 Through 2013–2014," table 1, Centers for Disease Control and Prevention, http://www .cdc.gov/nchs/data/hestat/obesity_adult_13_14/obesity_adult_13_14 .htm#Figure, accessed 12/2/16.

32   N. Howlader et al. (eds.), "SEER Cancer Statistics Review, 1975–2013."

33   "SEER Stat Fact Sheets: Cancer of Any Site," National Cancer Institute, http://seer.cancer.gov/statfacts/html/all.html, accessed November 28, 2016.

34   P. A. Heidenreich et al., "Forecasting the Future of Cardiovascular Disease in the United States," *Circulation*, 123, no. 8, (2011): 933-944, DOI: 10.1161 /CIR.0b013e31820a55f5.

35   P. Leren, "The Effect of Plasma-Cholesterol-Lowering Diet in Male Survivors of Myocardial Infarction: A Controlled Clinical Trial," *Bulletin of the New York Academy of Medicine*, 44, no. 8 (1968):1012–20.

36   S. Dayton et al., "A Controlled Clinical Trial of a Diet High in Unsaturated Fat in Preventing Complications of Atherosclerosis," *Circulation*, 40 (1969): II-1-II-63, DOI: 10.1161/01.CIR.40.1S2.II-1.

37   I. D. Frantz et al., "Test of effect of lipid lowering by diet on cardiovascular risk. The Minnesota Coronary Survey," *Arteriosclerosis*, 9, no. 1, (January–February 1989):129–35, DOI: 10.1161/01.ATV.9.1.129.

38   O. Turpeinen et al., "Dietary Prevention of Coronary Heart Disease: The Finnish Mental Hospital Study," *International Journal of Epidemiology*, 9, no. 2 (1979): 99–118, DOI: 10.1093/ije/8.2.99.

39   "Controlled Trial of Soya-Bean Oil in Myocardial Infarction," *The Lancet*, 292, no. 7570 (1968): 693–700, DOI: 10.1016/S0140-6736(68)90746-0.

40   "Multiple Risk Factor Intervention Trial Group: Public Annual Report, Multiple Risk Factor Intervention Trial, June 30, 1975 to July 1, 1976," *Journal of the American Medical Association*, 248, no. 12 (1982): 1465–77, https://clinicaltrials .gov/ct2/show/NCT00000487, accessed 12/2/16.

41   P. W. Siri-Tarino et al., "Meta-analysis of Prospective Cohort Studies Evaluating the Association of Saturated Fat with Cardiovascular Disease," *American Journal of Clinical Nutrition*, 91, no. 3 (2010): 535–46, DOI:10.3945/ajcn.2009.27725.

42   R. Chowdhury et al., "Association of Dietary, Circulating, and Supplement Fatty Acids With Coronary Risk: A Systematic Review and Meta-analysis," *Annals of Internal Medicine*, 160 (2014): 398–406, DOI: 10.7326/M13-1788.

43   De Souza et al., "Intake of Saturated and Trans Unsaturated Fatty Acids and Risk of All Cause Mortality, Cardiovascular Disease, and Type 2 Diabetes."

44   C. E. Ramsden et al., "Use of Dietary Linoleic Acid for Secondary Prevention of Coronary Heart Disease and Death: Evaluation of Recovered Data From the Sydney Diet Heart Study and Updated Meta-analysis," *BMJ*, 346 (2013): DOI: 0.1136/bmj.e8707.

45   Ibid.

46   M. A. Austin et al., "Low-Density Lipoprotein Subclass Patterns and Risk of Myocardial Infarction," *Journal of the American Medical Association*, 260, no. 13 (1988):1917–21, DOI: 10.1001/jama.1988.03410130125037.

47   D. M. Dreon et al., "Change in Dietary Saturated Fat Intake Is Correlated with Change in Mass of Large Low-Density-Lipoprotein Particles in Men," *American Journal of Clinical Nutrition*, 67, no. 5 (1998): 828–36, accessed 12/2/16.

48   K. Gunnars, "Saturated Fat, Good or Bad?" Authority Nutrition, https:// authoritynutrition.com/saturated-fat-good-or-bad/, accessed 12/2/16.

49   P. W. Siri-Tarino et al., "Saturated Fat, Carbohydrate, and Cardiovascular Disease," *American Journal of Clinical Nutrition*, 91, no. 3 (2010): 502–9, DOI: 10.3945/ajcn.2008.26285.

Chapter 2

1   L. Cordain, "The Nutritional Characteristics of a Contemporary Diet Based Upon Paleolithic Food Groups," *Journal of the American Nutraceutical Association*, 5, no. 5, (2002): 15–24.

2   J. J. Meidenbauer, P. Mukherjee, and T. N. Seyfried, "The Glucose Ketone Index Calculator: A Simple Tool to Monitor Therapeutic Efficacy for Metabolic Management of Brain Cancer," *Nutrition & Metabolism*, vol. 12 (2015):12. DOI:10.1186/s12986-015-0009-2.

3   R. Agrawal and F. Gomez-Pinilla, "'Metabolic Syndrome' in the Brain: Deficiency in Omega-3 Fatty Acid Exacerbates Dysfunctions in Insulin Receptor Signalling and Cognition," *The Journal of Physiology*, 590, no. 10, (2012): 2485, DOI: 10.1113/jphysiol.2012.230078.

4   J. R. Ifland et al., "Refined Food Addiction: A Classic Substance Use Disorder," *Medical Hypotheses*, 72, no. 5, (May 2009): 518–26, DOI: 10.1016/j .mehy.2008.11.035.

5   T. R. Nansel et al., "Greater Food Reward Sensitivity Is Associated with More Frequent Intake of Discretionary Foods in a Nationally Representative Sample

of Young Adults," *Frontiers in Nutrition*, 3, no. 33, 8/18/2016, DOI: 10.3389 /fnut.2016.00033.

6   S. D. Phinney and J. S. Volek, *The Art and Science of Low-Carbohydrate Living* (Miami, FL: Beyond Obesity LLC, 2011), 10.

7   G. D. Maurer, et al., "Differential Utilization of Ketone Bodies by Neurons and Glioma Cell Lines: a Rationale for Ketogenic Diet as Experimental Glioma Therapy," *BMC Cancer* 11 (2011): 315, DOI:10.1186/1471-2407-11-315.

8   R. Sender, S. Fuchs, and R. Milo, "Revised Estimates for the Number of Human and Bacteria Cells in the Body," *PLoS Biology*, 14, no. 8 (2016): e1002533, DOI:10.1371/journal.pbio.1002533.

9   R. Rosedale, "Life, Death, Food and the Disease of Aging," presented at the American Academy of Anti-Aging in Orlando, Florida, 2011.

10   C. E. Forsythe et al., "Comparison of Low Fat and Low Carbohydrate Diets on Circulation Fatty Acid Composition and Markers of Inflammation," *Lipids*, 43, no. 1 *(*2008): 65–77, DOI: 10.1007/s11745-007-3132-7.

11   S. McKenzie, "Yoshinori Ohsumi Wins Nobel Prize for Medical Research on Cells," CNN.com, October 3, 2016, http://www.cnn.com/2016/10/03/health /nobel-prize-2016-physiology-medicine-yoshinori-ohsumi/, accessed 12/2/16.

12   K. J. Bough et al., "Mitochondrial Biogenesis in the Anticonvulsant Mechanism of the Ketogenic Diet," *Annals of Neurology*, 60 (2006): 223–35, DOI:10.1002 /ana.20899.

13   P. J. Cox, K. Clarke, "Acute Nutritional Ketosis: Implications for Exercise Performance and Metabolism," *Extreme Physiology & Medicine*, 3 (2014): 1, DOI: 10.1186/2046-7648-3-17.

14   O. E. Owen et al., "Liver and Kidney Metabolism During Prolonged Starvation," *Journal of Clinical Investigation*, 48, no. 3 (1969): 574–83.

15   M. Akram, "A Focused Review of the Role of Ketone Bodies in Health and Disease," *Journal of Medicinal Food*, 16, no. 11 (November 2013): 965–67, DOI: 10.1089/jmf.2012.2592.

16   Ibid.

17   Phinney and Volek, *The Art and Science of Low-Carbohydrate Living*, 10.

18   Interview with Jeff Volek, Ph.D., http://articles.mercola.com/sites/articles /archive/2016/01/31/high-fat-low-carb-diet-benefits.aspx, accessed 12/2/16.

19   J. C. Newman and E. Verdin, "β-hydroxybutyrate: Much More Than a Metabolite," *Diabetes Research and Clinical Practice*, 106, no. 2 (2014): 173–81, DOI: 10.1016/j.diabres.2014.08.009.

20   A. Paoli et al., "Ketogenic Diet in Neuromuscular and Neurodegenerative Diseases," *BioMed Research International*, 2014 (2014), DOI:10.1155/2014/474296.

21   M. A. McNally and A. L. Hartman, "Ketone Bodies in Epilepsy," *Journal of Neurochemistry*, 121, no. 1 (2012): 28–35, DOI: 10.1111/j.1471 -4159.2012.07670.x.

22   J. Moore, *Keto Clarity* (Victory Belt Publishing, 2014), 58.

23   A. J. Brown, "Low-Carb Diets, Fasting and Euphoria: Is There a Link between Ketosis and Gamma-hydroxybutyrate (GHB)?" *Medical Hypotheses*, 68, no. 2 (2007): 268–71, DOI: 10.1016/j.mehy.2006.07.043.

Chapter 3

1   E. L. Knight et al., "The Impact of Protein Intake on Renal Function Decline in Women with Normal Renal Function or Mild Renal Insufficiency," *Annals of Internal Medicine*, 138. no. 6 (2003): 460–67, DOI: 10.7326/0003-4819-138-6 -200303180-00009.

2   M. I. Frisard et al., "Effect of 6-Month Calorie Restriction on Biomarkers of Longevity, Metabolic Adaptation, and Oxidative Stress in Overweight Individuals: A Randomized Controlled Trial," http://jamanetwork.com /journals/jama/fullarticle/1108368.

3   M. E. Levine et al., "Low Protein Intake Is Associated with a Major Reduction in IGF-1, Cancer, and Overall Mortality in the 65 and Younger but Not Older Population," *Cell Metabolism*, 19, no. 3 (2014): 407–17, DOI: 10.1016/j .cmet.2014.02.006.

4   J. Guevara-Aguirre et al., "Growth Hormone Receptor Deficiency Is Associated With a Major Reduction in Pro-aging Signaling, Cancer and Diabetes in Humans," *Science Translational Medicine*, 3, no. 70 (2011): 70, DOI: 10.1126 /scitranslmed.3001845.

5   S. I. A. Apelo and D. W. Lamming, "Rapamycin: An InhibiTOR of Aging Emerges From the Soil of Easter Island," *Journal of Gerontology*, 71, no. 7 (2016): 841-849, DOI: 10.1093/gerona/glw090.

6   S. M. Solon-Biet et al., "The Ratio of Macronutrients, Not Caloric Intake, Dictates Cardiometabolic Health, Aging, and Longevity in Ad Libitum-Fed Mice," *Cell Metabolism*, 19, no. 3 (2014): 418–30, DOI: 10.1016/j .cmet.2014.02.009.

Chapter 4

1   "Ferritin: The Test," American Association for Clinical Chemistry, https:// labtestsonline.org/understanding/analytes/ferritin/tab/test/, accessed May 9, 2016.

2   E. D. Weinberg, "The Hazards of Iron Loading," *Metallomics*, 2, no. 11 (November, 2010):732–40, DOI: 10.1039/c0mt00023j.

3   M. D. Beaton and P. C. Adams, "Treatment of Hyperferritinemia," *Annals of Hepatology*, 11, no. 3 (2012): 294–300, PMID: 22481446.

4   G. Ortíz-Estrada et al., "Iron-Saturated Lactoferrin and Pathogenic Protozoa: Could This Protein Be an Iron Source for Their Parasitic Style of Life?" *Future Microbiology*, 7, no. 1 (2012): 149–64, DOI: 10.2217/fmb.11.140.

5   D. J. Fleming et al., "Dietary Factors Associated with the Risk of High Iron Stores in the Elderly Framingham Heart Study Cohort," *American Journal of Clinical Nutrition*, 76, no. 6 (2002): 1375–84, PMID: 12450906.

6   T. Iwasaki et al., "Serum Ferritin Is Associated with Visceral Fat Area and Subcutaneous Fat Area," *Diabetes Care*, 28, no. 10 (2005): 2486–91, PMID: 16186284.

7   S. K. Park et al., "Association between Serum Ferritin Levels and the Incidence of Obesity in Korean Men: A Prospective Cohort Study," *Endocrine Journal*, 61, no. 3 (2014): 215–24, DOI: 10.1507/endocrj.EJ13-0173.

8   Ibid.

9   J. M. Fernandez-Real et al., "Serum Ferritin as a Component of the Insulin Resistance Syndrome," *Diabetes Care*, 21, no. 1 (1998): 62–68, DOI: 10.2337 /diacare.21.1.62.

10   J. Montonen et al., "Body Iron Stores and Risk of Type 2 Diabetes: Results from the European Prospective Investigation into Cancer and Nutrition (EPIC)-Potsdam Study," *Diabetologia*, 55, no. 10 (2012): 2613–21, DOI: 10.1007 /s00125-012-2633-y.

11   J. M. Fernández-Real, A. López-Bermejo, and W. Ricart, "Iron Stores, Blood Donation, and Insulin Sensitivity and Secretion," *Clinical Chemistry*, 51, no. 7 (June 2005): 1201–5, DOI: 10.1373/clinchem.2004.046847.

12   B. J. Van Lenten et al., "Lipid-Induced Changes in Intracellular Iron Homeostasis in Vitro and in Vivo," *Journal of Clinical Investigation*, 95, no. 5 (1995): 2104–10, DOI: 10.1172/JCI117898.

13   N. Stadler, R. A. Lindner, and M. J. Davies, "Direct Detection and Quantification of Transition Metal Ions in Human Atherosclerotic Plaques: Evidence for the Presence of Elevated Levels of Iron and Copper," *Arteriosclerosis, Thrombosis, and Vascular Biology*, 24 (2004): 949–54, DOI: 10.1161/01.ATV.0000124892.90999.cb.

14   W. B. Kannel et al., "Menopause and Risk of Cardiovascular Disease: The Framingham Study," *Annals of Internal Medicine*, 85 (1976): 447–52, DOI: 10.7326/0003-4819-85-4-447.

15   M. A. Lovell et al., "Copper, Iron and Zinc in Alzheimer's Disease Senile Plaques," *Journal of the Neurological Sciences*, 158, no. 1 (June 11, 1998): 47–52, DOI: 10.1016/S0022-510X(98)00092-6.

16   K. Jellinger et al., "Brain Iron and Ferritin in Parkinson's and Alzheimer's diseases," *Journal of Neural Transmission*, 2 (1990): 327, DOI: 10.1007 /BF02252926.

17   G. Bartzokis et al., "Brain Ferritin Iron as a Risk Factor for Age at Onset in Neurodegenerative Diseases," *Annals of the New York Academy of Sciences*, 1012, (2004): 224–36, DOI: 10.1196/annals.1306.019.

18   S. Ayton et al., "Ferritin Levels in the Cerebrospinal Fluid Predict Alzheimer's Disease Outcomes and Are Regulated by APOE," *Nature Communications*, 6 (2015): 6760, DOI: 10.1038/ncomms7760.

19   W. Z. Zhu et al., "Quantitative MR Phase-Corrected Imaging to Investigate Increased Brain Iron Deposition of Patients with Alzheimer's Disease," *Radiology*, 253 (2009): 497–504, DOI: 10.1148/radiol.2532082324.

20   A. A. Alkhateeb and J. R. Connor, "The Significance of Ferritin in Cancer: Anti-Oxidation, Inflammation and Tumorigenesis," *Biochimica et Biophysica Acta*, 1836, no. 2 (Dec 2013):245–54, DOI: 10.1016/j.bbcan.2013.07.002.

21   J. I. Wurzelmann et al., "Iron Intake and the Risk of Colorectal Cancer," *Cancer Epidemiology, Biomarkers and Prevention*, 5, no. 7 (July 1, 1996): 503–7. PMID: 8827353.

22   Y. Deugnier, "Iron and Liver Cancer," *Alcohol*, 30, no. 2 (2003): 145–50.

23   L. R. Zacharski et al., "Decreased Cancer Risk after Iron Reduction in Patients with Peripheral Arterial Disease: Results from a Randomized Trial," *JNCI:*

Journal of National Cancer Institute, 100, no. 14 (2008): 996–1002, DOI: 10.1093/jnci/djn209.

24   L. Valenti et al., "Association between Iron Overload and Osteoporosis in Patients with Hereditary Hemochromatosis," *Osteoporosis International*, 20, no. 4 (April, 2009): 549–55, DOI: 10.1007/s00198-008-0701-4.

25   "Hemochromatosis," National Institute of Diabetes and Digestive and Kidney Disease (2016), http://www.niddk.nih.gov/health-information/health-topics /liver-disease/hemochromatosis/Pages/facts.aspx, accessed May 9, 2016.

26   "Welcome," Iron Disorders Institute (2016) http://www.hemochromatosis .org/#symptoms, accessed May 9, 2016.

27   "Serum Iron Test," MedlinePlus Medical Encyclopedia (2016), https://www .nlm.nih.gov/medlineplus/ency/article/003488.htm, accessed May 9, 2016.

28   "TIBC, UIBC, and Transferrin Test: Iron Binding Capacity; IBC; Serum Iron-Binding Capacity; Siderophilin; Total Iron Binding Capacity; Unsaturated Iron Binding Capacity," Lab Tests Online (2016), https://labtestsonline.org /understanding/analytes/tibc/tab/test/, accessed May 9, 2016.

29   L. Zacharski, "Ferrotoxic Disease: The Next Great Public Health Challenge," *Clinical Chemistry*, 60, no. 11 (November 2014): 1362–4, DOI: 10.1373 /clinchem.2014.231266.

30   P. Mangan, *Dumping Iron: How to Ditch This Secret Killer and Reclaim Your Health*, Phalanx Press, 2016, locations 308–12.

31   Ibid., locations 1353–56.

32   Ibid., locations 1609–12.

33   Ibid., locations 416–18.

34   Ibid., locations 428–31.

35   Ibid., locations 582–95.

Chapter 5

1   C. Manisha Chandalia et al., "Beneficial Effects of High Dietary Fiber Intake in Patients with Type 2 Diabetes Mellitus," *New England Journal of Medicine*, 342 (2000):1392–98, DOI: 10.1056/NEJM200005113421903.

2   M. Wien et al., "A Randomized 3x3 Crossover Study to Evaluate the Effect of Hass Avocado Intake on Post-ingestive Satiety, Glucose and Insulin Levels, and Subsequent Energy Intake in Overweight Adults," *Nutrition Journal*, 12, (2013): 155, DOI: 10.1186/1475-2891-12-155.

3   "Potassium," University of Maryland Medical Center, http://umm.edu/health /medical/altmed/supplement/potassium, accessed November 28, 2016.

4   M. E. Cogswell et al., "Sodium and Potassium Intakes among U.S. Adults: NHANES 2003–2008," *The American Journal of Clinical Nutrition*, 96, no. 3 (2012): 647–57, DOI: 10.3945/ajcn.112.034413.

5   M. L. Dreher and A. J. Davenport, "Hass Avocado Composition and Potential Health Effects," *Critical Reviews in Food Science and Nutrition*, 53, no. 7 (2013): 738–50, DOI: 10.1080/10408398.2011.556759.

6   R. E. Kopec et al., "Avocado Consumption Enhances Human Postprandial Provitamin A Absorption and Conversion from a Novel High–β-Carotene Tomato Sauce and from Carrots," *Journal of Nutrition*, 8 (2014), DOI: 10.3945 /jn.113.187674.

7   N. Z. Unlu et al., "Carotenoid Absorption from Salad and Salsa by Humans Is Enhanced by the Addition of Avocado or Avocado Oil," *Journal of Nutrition*, 135, no. 3 (2005): 431–36.

8   E. A. Lee et al., "Targeting Mitochondria with Avocatin B Induces Selective Leukemia Cell Death," *Cancer Research*, 75, no. 12 (June 15 2015): 2478–88, DOI: 10.1158/0008-5472.CAN-14-2676.

9   M. Notarnicola et al., "Effects of Olive Oil Polyphenols on Fatty Acid Synthase Gene Expression and Activity in Human Colorectal Cancer Cells," *Genes & Nutrition*, 6, no. 1 (2011): 63–69, DOI: 10.1007/s12263-010-0177-7.

10   A. Cañuelo et al., "Tyrosol, a Main Phenol Present in Extra Virgin Olive Oil, Increases Lifespan and Stress Resistance in Caenorhabditis Elegans," *Mechanisms of Ageing and Development*, 133, no. 8 (2012): 563–74, DOI: 10.1016/j.mad.2012.07.004.

11   A. H. Rahmani, A. S. Albutti, and S. M. Aly, "Therapeutics Role of Olive Fruits/ Oil in the Prevention of Diseases via Modulation of Anti-Oxidant, Anti-Tumour and Genetic Activity," *International Journal of Clinical and Experimental Medicine*, 7, no. 4 (2014): 799–808, PMID: 24955148.

12   J. M. Fernández-Real et al., "A Mediterranean Diet Enriched with Olive Oil Is Associated with Higher Serum Total Osteocalcin Levels in Elderly Men at High Cardiovascular Risk," *The Journal of Clinical Endocrinology and Metabolism*, 97, no. 10 (2012): 3792–98, DOI: 10.1210/jc.2012-2221.

13   O. García-Martínez et al., "Phenolic Compounds in Extra Virgin Olive Oil Stimulate Human Osteoblastic Cell Proliferation," *PLoS ONE*, 11, no. 3 (2016): e0150045, DOI: 10.1371/journal.pone.0150045.

14   "Food Fraud Database," U.S. Pharmacopeial Convention, http://www .foodfraud.org/, accessed December 6, 2016.

15   "Sardines," The George Mateljan Foundation, http://www.whfoods.com /genpage.php?tname=foodspice&dbid=147, accessed November 28, 2016.

16   K. Warner, W. Timme, B. Lowell, and M. Hirshfield, "Oceana Study Reveals Seafood Fraud Nationwide," February 2013, http://usa.oceana.org/sites/default /files/National_Seafood_Fraud_Testing_Results_Highlights_FINAL.pdf, accessed December 8, 2016.

17   http://articles.mercola.com/sites/articles/archive/2015/05/13/seafood-shrimp -industry-fraud.aspx#_edn1.

18   http://articles.mercola.com/sites/articles/archive/2015/05/13/seafood-shrimp -industry-fraud.aspx#_edn2.

19   http://articles.mercola.com/sites/articles/archive/2015/05/13/seafood-shrimp -industry-fraud.aspx#_edn3.

20   http://articles.mercola.com/sites/articles/archive/2015/05/13/seafood-shrimp -industry-fraud.aspx#_edn15.

21   http://articles.mercola.com/sites/articles/archive/2015/05/13/seafood-shrimp -industry-fraud.aspx#_edn16.

22 N. Greenfield, "The Smart Seafood Buying Guide," https://www.nrdc.org
    /stories/smart-seafood-buying-guide, accessed November 28, 2016.

23 M. Neuhouser et al., "Food and Nutrient Intakes, and Health: Current Status
    and Trends," Dietary Guidelines Advisory Committee, https://health.gov
    /dietaryguidelines/2015-BINDER/meeting7/docs/DGAC-Meeting-7-SC-1.pdf,
    accessed December 8, 2016.

24 B. S. Luh, W. S. Wong, and N. E. El-Shimi, "Effect of Processing on Some
    Chemical Constituents of Pistachio Nuts," *Journal of Food Quality*, 5 (1982):
    33–41, DOI: 10.1111/j.1745-4557.1982.tb00954.x.

25 S. M. Solon-Biet et al., "The Ratio of Macronutrients, Not Caloric Intake,
    Dictates Cardiometabolic Health, Aging, and Longevity in Ad Libitum-Fed
    Mice," *Cell Metabolism*, 19, no. 3 (418–30), DOI: 10.1016/j.cmet.2014.02.009.

26 A. Villalvilla et al., "Lipid Transport and Metabolism in Healthy and
    Osteoarthritic Cartilage," *International Journal of Molecular Sciences*, 14, no. 10
    (2013): 20793-20808, DOI: 10.3390/ijms141020793.

Chapter 6

1   J. A. Vasquez and J. E. Janosky, "Validity of Bioelectrical-Impedance Analysis in
    Measuring Changes in Body Mass During Weight Reduction," *American Journal
    of Clinical Nutrition*, 54, no. 6 (1991): 970–5, PMID 1957829.

Chapter 7

1   A. G. Bergqvist et al., "Fasting Versus Gradual Initiation of the Ketogenic Diet:
    A Prospective, Randomized Clinical Trial of Efficacy," *Epilepsia*, 46, no. 11
    (November 2005): 1810–19, DOI: 10.1111/j.1528-1167.2005.00282.x.

Chapter 8

1   "A Daily Walk Can Add Seven Years to Your Life," *The Independent*, http://www
    .independent.co.uk/life-style/health-and-families/health-news/a-daily-walk-can
    -add-seven-year-to-your-life-10478821.html, accessed November 28, 2016.

Chapter 9

1   C. Newell et al., "Ketogenic Diet Modifies the Gut Microbiota in a Murine
    Model of Autism Spectrum Disorder," *Molecular Autism*, 7, no. 1 (2016): 37, DOI:
    10.1186/s13229-016-0099-3.

2   S. B. Eaton and M. Konner, "Paleolithic Nutrition—A Consideration of Its
    Nature and Current Implications," *New England Journal of Medicine*, 312 (1985):
    283–289, DOI: 10.1056/NEJM198501313120505.

3   D. Piovesan et al., "The Human 'Magnesome': Detecting Magnesium
    Binding Sites on Human Proteins" *BMC Bioinformatics*, 13, no. 14 supplement
    (2012):S10, DOI: 10.1186/1471-2105-13-S14-S10.

4   "Magnesium: Fact Sheet for Health Professionals," U.S. Department of Health
    and Human Services, https://ods.od.nih.gov/factsheets/Magnesium
    -HealthProfessional/, accessed November 28, 2016.

Chapter 10

1   "Overweight and Obesity Statistics," U.S. Department of Health and Human Services, https://www.niddk.nih.gov/health-information/health-statistics /Pages/overweight-obesity-statistics.aspx, accessed November 28, 2016.

2   S. Gill and S. Panda, "A Smartphone App Reveals Erratic Diurnal Eating Patterns in Humans that Can Be Modulated for Health Benefits," *Cell Metabolism*, 22, no. 5 (November 3, 2015): 789–98, DOI: 10.1016/j .cmet.2015.09.005.

3   "Autophagy Key to Restoring Function in Old Muscle Stem Cells," Sens Research Foundation, https://www.fightaging.org/archives/2016/01/autophagy -key-to-restoring-function-in-old-muscle-stem-cells/, accessed November 28, 2016.

4   A. M. Johnstone et al., "Effect of an Acute Fast on Energy Compensation and Feeding Behaviour in Lean Men and Women," *International Journal of Obesity*, 26, no 12 (2002): 1623-8, DOI: 10.1038/sj.ijo.0802151.

5   Gill and Panda, "A Smartphone App Reveals Erratic Diurnal Eating Patterns in Humans."

6   V. K. M. Halagappa et al., "Intermittent Fasting and Caloric Restriction Ameliorate Age-Related Behavioral Deficits in the Triple-Transgenic Mouse Model of Alzheimer's Disease," *Neurobiology of Disease*, 26, no. 1 (2007): 212–20, DOI: 10.1016/j.nbd.2006.12.019.

7   A. M. Stranahan and M. P. Mattson, "Recruiting Adaptive Cellular Stress Responses for Successful Brain Ageing," *Nature Reviews Neuroscience*, 13, no. 3 (March 2012): 209–16, DOI: 10.1038/nrn3151.

8   S. Brandhorst et al., "A Periodic Diet That Mimics Fasting Promotes Multi-System Regeneration, Enhanced Cognitive Performance, and Healthspan," *Cell Metabolism*, 22, no. 1 (July 7, 2015): 86–99, DOI: 10.1016/j.cmet.2015.05.012.

9   K. Varady et al., "Alternate Day Fasting for Weight Loss in Normal Weight and Overweight Subjects: A Randomized Controlled Trial," *Nutrition Journal*, 12 (2013): 146, DOI: 10.1186/1475-2891-12-146.

10 I. Ahmet et al., "Chronic Alternate Day Fasting Results in Reduced Diastolic Compliance and Diminished Systolic Reserve in Rats," *Journal of Cardiac Failure*, 16, no. 10 (2010):843-853, DOI: 10.1016/j.cardfail.2010.05.007.

11 C. R. Marinac et al., "Prolonged Nightly Fasting and Breast Cancer Prognosis," *Journal of the American Medical Association Oncology*, 2, no. 8 (2016):1049–55, DOI: 10.1001/jamaoncol.2016.0164.

12 R. Pamplona, "Mitochondrial DNA Damage and Animal Longevity: Insights from Comparative Studies," *Journal of Aging Research*, 2011 (2011): DOI: 10.4061/2011/807108.

13 P. Sonksen and J. Sonksen, "Insulin: Understanding Its Action in Health and Disease," *British Journal of Anaesthesia*, 85, no. 1 (2000): 69–79, DOI: 10.1093 /bja/85.1.69.

14 M. J. Wargovich and J. E. Cunningham, "Diet, Individual Responsiveness and Cancer Prevention," *The Journal of Nutrition*, 133 (July 2003): 2400S–2403S, PMID 12840215.

15   M. V. Chakravarthy and F. W. Booth, "Eating, Exercise, and 'Thrifty'
     Genotypes: Connecting the Dots toward an Evolutionary Understanding of
     Modern Chronic Diseases," *Journal of Applied Physiology*, 96, no. 1 (2004): 3–10,
     DOI:10.1152/japplphysiol.00757.2003.

16   V. D. Longo and M. P. Mattson, "Fasting: Molecular Mechanisms and Clinical
     Applications," *Cell Metabolism*, 19, no. 2 (2014):181–92, DOI:10.1016/j
     .cmet.2013.12.008.

Chapter 11

1   G. Chevalier et al., "Earthing: Health Implications of Reconnecting the Human
    Body to the Earth's Surface Electrons," *Journal of Environmental and Public
    Health*, 2012, (2012), DOI: 10.1155/2012/291541.

2   J. L. Oschman, G. Chevalier, and R. Brown, "The Effects of Grounding
    (Earthing) on Inflammation, the Immune Response, Wound Healing, and
    Prevention and Treatment of Chronic Inflammatory and Autoimmune Diseases,"
    Journal of Inflammation Research, 8 (2015): 83–96, DOI: 10.2147/JIR.S69656.

3   D. Z. Kochan et al., "Circadian Disruption and Breast Cancer: An Epigenetic
    Link?," *Oncotarget*, 6, no. 19 (2015): 16866–16682. DOI:10.18632
    /oncotarget.4343.

4   M. Dunbar and R. Melton, "The Lowdown on Light: Good vs. Bad, and Its
    Connection to AMD," *Review of Optometry*, https://www.reviewofoptometry
    .com/ce/the-lowdown-on-blue-light-good-vs-bad-and-its-connection-to-
    amd-109744, accessed November 28, 2016.

5   D. Peretti et al., "RBM3 Mediates Structural Plasticity and Protective Effects
    of Cooling in Neurodegeneration," *Nature*, 518, no. 7538 (2015):236–39, DOI:
    10.1038/nature14142.

Appendix A

1   H. H. Kwon et al., "Clinical and Histological Effect of a Low Glycaemic
    Load Diet in Treatment of Acne Vulgaris in Korean Patients: A Randomized,
    Controlled Trial." *Acta Dermato Venereologica*, 92, no. 3 (May 2012): 241–46,
    DOI: 10.2340/00015555-1346.

2   L. Knott et al., "Regulation of Osteoarthritis by Omega-3 (n-3) Polyunsaturated
    Fatty Acids in a Naturally Occurring Model of Disease," *Osteoarthritis Cartilage*,
    19, no. 9 (September 2011): 1150–57, DOI: 10.1016/j.joca.2011.06.005.

3   L. Cordain et al., "Acne Vulgaris: A Disease of Western Civilization," *Archives of
    Dermatology*, 138, no. 12 (December 2002): 1584–0, DOI: 10.1001
    /archderm.138.12.1584.

4   R. N. Smith et al., "A Low-Glycemic-Load Diet Improves Symptoms in Acne
    Vulgaris Patients: A Randomized Controlled Trial," *American Journal of Clinical
    Nutrition*, 86, no. 1 (July 2007): 107–115.

5   Kwon et al., "Clinical and Histological Effect of a Low Glycaemic Load Diet in
    Treatment of Acne Vulgaris in Korean Patients."

6   S. N. Mahmood and W.P. Bowe, "Diet and Acne Update: Carbohydrates Emerge
    as the Main Culprit," *Journal of Drugs in Dermatology*, 13, no. 4, (April 2014):
    428–35.

7   "2015 Alzheimer's Disease Facts and Figures," Alzheimer's Association, https://
     www.alz.org/facts/downloads/facts_figures_2015.pdf, accessed November 28,
     2016.

8   World Health Organization. "Dementia: a Public Health Priority" (Geneva,
     SUI: World Health Organization, 2012), PMID: 19712582.

9   B. D. James et al., "Contribution of Alzheimer Disease to Mortality in the
     United States," *Neurology*, published online before print March 5, 2014, DOI:
     10.1212/WNL.0000000000000240.

10   V. R. Bitra, D. Rapaka, and A. Akula, "Prediabetes and Alzheimer's Disease,"
     Indian Journal of Pharmaceutical Sciences, 77, no. 5 (2015): 511–14.

11   S. M. de la Monte, "Insulin Resistance and Alzheimer's Disease," *BMB Reports*,
     42, no. 8 (2009): 475–81.

12   R. O. Roberts et al., "Relative Intake of Macronutrients Impacts Risk of Mild
     Cognitive Impairment or Dementia," *Journal of Alzheimer's Disease*, 32, no. 2
     (2012), 329–39. DOI: 10.3233/JAD-2012-120862.

13   S. T. Henderson et al., "Study of the Ketogenic Agent AC-1202 in Mild to
     Moderate Alzheimer's Disease: A Randomized, Double-Blind, Placebo-
     Controlled, Multicenter Trial," *Nutrition & Metabolism*, 6 (2009): 31. DOI:
     10.1186/1743-7075-6-31, PMID: 19664276.

14   J. Yao and R. D. Brinton, "Targeting Mitochondrial Bioenergetics for
     Alzheimer's Prevention and Treatment," *Current Pharmaceutical Design*, 17, no.
     31, (2011): 3474–79, PMID: 21902662.

15   J. M. Hootman et al., "Updated Projected Prevalence of Self-Reported Doctor-
     Diagnosed Arthritis and Arthritis-Attributable Activity Limitation Among US
     Adults, 2015–2040." *Arthritis & Rheumatololgy*, 68, no. 7 (July 2016):1582–87,
     DOI: 10.1002/art.39692.

16   Knott et al., "Regulation of Osteoarthritis by Omega-3 (n-3) Polyunsaturated
     Fatty Acids in a Naturally Occurring Model of Disease."

17   Y. M. Bastiaansen-Jenniskens et al., "Monounsaturated and Saturated, but
     Not n-6 Polyunsaturated Fatty Acids Decrease Cartilage Destruction under
     Inflammatory Conditions: A Preliminary Study." *Cartilage*, 4 no. 4 (2013),
     321–28. DOI: 10.1177/1947603513494401.

18   D. N. Ruskin, M. Kawamura, and S. A. Masino, "Reduced Pain and
     Inflammation in Juvenile and Adult Rats Fed a Ketogenic Diet," *PLoS ONE*, 4,
     no. 12 (2009): e8349, DOI:10.1371/journal.pone.0008349.

19   S. A. Masino and D. N. Ruskin, "Ketogenic Diets and Pain," *Journal of Child
     Neurology*, 28, no. 8 (2013): 993–1001. DOI: 10.1177/0883073813487595.

20   "Vital Signs: Preventable Deaths from Heart Disease & Stroke," Centers for
     Disease Control and Prevention, http://www.cdc.gov/dhdsp/vital_signs.htm,
     accessed November 28, 2016.

21   B. Hoogwerf et al., "Blood Glucose Concentrations ≤125 mg/dl and Coronary
     Heart Disease Risk,"*American Journal of Cardiology*, 89, no. 5, (2002): 596–99,
     DOI: 10.1016/S0002-9149(01)02302-5.

22   N. V. Dhurandhar and D. Thomas, "The Link between Dietary Sugar Intake
     and Cardiovascular Disease Mortality: An Unresolved Question," *Journal of the
     American Medical Association*, 313, no. 9 (2015): 959–60. DOI:10.1001
     /jama.2014.18267, accessed 12/2/16.

23   Q. Yang et al., "Added Sugar Intake and Cardiovascular Diseases Mortality Among US Adults," *JAMA Internal Medicine*, 174, no. 4 (2014), 516–24, DOI: 10.1001/jamainternmed.2013.13563.

24   L. Schwingshackl et al., "Comparison of Effects of Long-Term Low-Fat vs High-Fat Diets on Blood Lipid Levels in Overweight or Obese Patients: A Systematic Review and Meta-Analysis." *Journal of the Academy of Nutrition and Dietetics*, 113, no. 12 (2013), 1640–61, DOI: 10.1016/j.jand.2013.07.010.

25   C. L. Gibson, A. N. Murphy, and S. P. Murphy, "Stroke Outcome in the Ketogenic State: A Systematic Review of the Animal Data," *Journal of Neurochemistry*, 123, no. 2 (2012), 52–57, DOI:10.1111/j.1471-4159.2012.07943.x.

26   "Epilepsy Fast Facts," Centers for Disease Control and Prevention, http://www.cdc.gov/epilepsy/basics/fast-facts.htm, accessed November 28, 2016.

27   J. W. Wheless, "History of the Ketogenic Diet," *Epilepsia*, 49, Suppl. 8 (November 2008): 3–5, DOI: 10.1111/j.1528-1167.2008.01821.x.

28   K. Martin et al., "Ketogenic Diet and Other Dietary Treatments for Epilepsy," *Cochrane Database of Systematic Reviews*, 2 (2016), DOI: 10.1002/14651858 .CD001903.pub3.

29   "What Is Fibromyalgia?," (November 2014), http://www.niams.nih.gov/.

30   Mayo Clinic, "Diseases and Conditions: Fibromyalgia," http://www.mayoclinic .org/diseases-conditions/fibromyalgia/basics/causes/con-20019243, accessed November 28, 2016.

31   Paper presented at the Annual Meeting of the American College of Nutrition in Orlando, Florida, October 2001.

32   M. Meeus et al., "The Role of Mitochondrial Dysfunctions Due to Oxidative and Nitrosative Stress in the Chronic Pain or Chronic Fatigue Syndromes and Fibromyalgia Patients: Peripheral and Central Mechanisms as Therapeutic Targets?" *Expert Opinion on Therapeutic Target*, 17, no. 9 (2013): 1081–89, DOI: 10.1517/14728222.2013.818657.

33   A. Ernst and J. Shelley-Tremblay, "Non-Ketogenic, Low Carbohydrate Diet Predicts Lower Affective Distress, Higher Energy Levels and Decreased Fibromyalgia Symptoms in Middle-Aged Females with Fibromyalgia Syndrome as Compared to the Western Pattern Diet," *Journal of Musculoskeletal Pain*, 21, no. 4 (2013): 365–70, DOI: 10.3109/10582452.2013.852649.

34   "GERD," American Gastroenterological Association, http://www.gastro.org /patient-care/conditions-diseases/gerd, accessed November 28, 2016.

35   "A Sunny Day in Pharmaland: The 2015 Pharma Report," Medical Marketing & Media, http://media.mmm-online.com/documents/119/pharma _report_2015_29732.pdf, accessed November 28, 2016.

36   Singh et al., "Weight Loss Can Lead to Resolution of Gastroesophageal Reflux Disease Symptoms: A Prospective Intervention Trial," *Obesity*, 21, no. 2 (2013), DOI: 10.1002/oby.20279.

37   G. L. Austin et al., "A Very Low-Carbohydrate Diet Improves Gastroesophageal Reflux and Its Symptoms," *Digestive Diseases and Sciences*, 51, no. 8 (August 2006): 1307–12, DOI: 10.1007/s10620-005-9027-7.

38   Singh et al., "Weight Loss Can Lead to Resolution of Gastroesophageal Reflux Disease Symptoms."

39 G. L. Austin et al., "A Very Low-Carbohydrate Diet Improves Symptoms and Quality of Life in Diarrhea-Predominant Irritable Bowel Syndrome," *Clinical Gastroenterology and Hepatology: The Official Clinical Practice Journal of the American Gastroenterological Association*, 7, no. 6 (2009): 706–08.e1. DOI: 10.1016/j.cgh.2009.02.023.

40 Z. Zheng et al., "Staple Foods Consumption and Irritable Bowel Syndrome in Japanese Adults: A Cross-Sectional Study," *PLoS ONE*, 10, no. 3 (2015): e0119097, DOI:10.1371/journal.pone.0119097.

41 "Migraine Statistics," Migraine.com, https://migraine.com/migraine-statistics/, accessed November 28, 2016.

42 PubMed.gov, https://www.ncbi.nlm.nih.gov/pubmed/?term=migraine+food+allergy, accessed November 28, 2016.

43 K. Alpay et al., "Diet Restriction in Migraine, Based on IgG Against Foods: A Clinical Double-blind, Randomised, Cross-over Trial," *Cephalalgia*, 30, no. 7 (2010): 829–37, DOI:10.1177/0333102410361404.

44 C. Di Lorenzo et al., "Migraine Improvement During Short Lasting Ketogenesis: A Proof-of-Concept Study," *European Journal of Neurology*, 22, no. 1 (2015):170–7, DOI: 10.1111/ene.12550.

45 C. Di Lorenzo et al., "Diet Transiently Improves Migraine in Two Twin Sisters: Possible Role of Ketogenesis?," *Functional Neurology*, 28, no. 4 (2013): 305–308.

46 K. L. Munger et al., "Vitamin D Intake and Incidence of Multiple Sclerosis," *Neurology*, 62, no. 1, (2004): 60–65, PMID:14718698.

47 D. Y. Kim et al., "Inflammation-Mediated Memory Dysfunction and Effects of a Ketogenic Diet in a Murine Model of Multiple Sclerosis," *PLoS ONE*, 7, no. 5 (2012): e35476, DOI: 10.1371/journal.pone.0035476.

48 M. Storoni and G. T. Plant, "The Therapeutic Potential of the Ketogenic Diet in Treating Progressive Multiple Sclerosis," *Multiple Sclerosis International*, 2015 (2015): 681289, DOI: 10.1155/2015/681289.

49 Ibid.

50 "Non-Alcoholic Fatty Liver Disease," American Liver Foundation, http://www.liverfoundation.org/abouttheliver/info/nafld/, accessed November 28, 2016.

51 S. S. Sundaram, "Pediatric Non-Alcoholic Fatty Liver Disease," American Liver Foundation, http://www.liverfoundation.org/chapters/rockymountain/doctorsnotes/pediatricnafld/, accessed November 28, 2016.

52 J. Ma et al., "Sugar-sweetened Beverage, Diet Soda, and Fatty Liver Disease in the Framingham Heart Study Cohorts," *Journal of Hepatology*, 63, no. 2 (2015): 462–69, DOI: 10.1016/j.jhep.2015.03.032.

53 J. D. Browning et al., "Short-term Weight Loss and Hepatic Triglyceride Reduction: Evidence of a Metabolic Advantage with Dietary Carbohydrate Restriction," *The American Journal of Clinical Nutrition*, 93, no. 5 (2011): 1048–52. DOI: 10.3945/ajcn.110.007674.

54 J. Pérez-Guisado and A. Muñoz-Serrano, "The Effect of the Spanish Ketogenic Mediterranean Diet on Nonalcoholic Fatty Liver Disease: A Pilot Study," *Journal of Medicinal Food*, 14, no. 7–8 (July–August 2011): 677-80, DOI: 10.1089/jmf.2011.0075.

55 D. Tendler et al., "The Effect of a Low-Carbohydrate, Ketogenic Diet on Nonalcoholic Fatty Liver Disease: A Pilot Study," *Digestive Diseases and Sciences*, 52, no. 2 (February, 2007): 589–93, DOI: 10.1007/s10620-006-9433-5.

56 P. Kennedy, "The Fat Drug." *The New York Times*, March 8, 2014, http://www .nytimes.com/2014/03/09/opinion/sunday/the-fat-drug.html?_r=0, accessed 12/2/16.

57 H.-Y. Kim et al., "Phosphatidylserine-dependent Neuroprotective Signaling Promoted by Docosahexaenoic Acid," *Prostaglandins, Leukotrienes, and Essential Fatty Acids*, 82, no. 4–6 (2010): 165–72, DOI:10.1016/j.plefa.2010.02.025.

58 H.-Y. Kim et al., "*N*-Docosahexaenoylethanolamide Promotes Development of Hippocampal Neurons," *The Biochemical Journal*, 435, no. 2 (2011): 327–36, DOI: 10.1042/BJ20102118.

59 R. Palacios-Pelaez, W. J. Lukiw, and N. G. Bazan, "Omega-3 Essential Fatty Acids Modulate Initiation and Progression of Neurodegenerative Disease," *Molecular Neurobiology*, 41, no. 2–3 (June 2010): 367-74, DOI: 10.1007/s12035 -010-8139-z.

60 Interview with J. J. Virgin, http://articles.mercola.com/sites/articles /archive/2014/02/09/fish-oil-brain-health.aspx, accessed 12/2/16.

61 S. Smith, "Fish Oil Helped Save Our Son," CNN, http://www.cnn .com/2012/10/19/health/fish-oil-brain-injuries/index.html, accessed 12/2/16.

62 M. L. Prins and J. H. Matsumoto, "The Collective Therapeutic Potential of Cerebral Ketone Metabolism in Traumatic Brain Injury," *Journal of Lipid Research*, 55, no. 12 (2014):2450–57, DOI: 10.1194/jlr.R046706.

63 H. Algattas and J. H. Huang, "Traumatic Brain Injury Pathophysiology and Treatments: Early, Intermediate, and Late Phases Post-Injury," *International Journal of Molecular Sciences*, 15, no. 1 (2014): 309–41, DOI: 10.3390 /ijms15010309.

64 Ibid.

65 M. L. Prins, L. S. Fujima, and D. A. Hovda, "Age-dependent Reduction of Cortical Contusion Volume by Ketones After Traumatic Brain Injury," *Journal of Neuroscience Research*, 82, no. 3 (November 1, 2005): 413–20, DOI: 10.1002 /jnr.20633.

66 Z. G. Hu et al., "The Protective Effect of the Ketogenic Diet on Traumatic Brain Injury-Induced Cell Death in Juvenile Rats," *Brain Injury*, 23, no. 5 (2009): 459–65, DOI: 10.1080/02699050902788469.

67 "National Diabetes Statistics Report, 2014," National Center for Chronic Disease Prevention and Health Promotion, http://www.cdc.gov/diabetes/pubs /statsreport14/national-diabetes-report-web.pdf, accessed 12/2/16.

68 "Diabetes Facts and Figures," International Diabetes Foundation, http://www .idf.org/about-diabetes/facts-figures, accessed November 28, 2016.

69 D. Dabelea et al., "Prevalence of Type 1 and Type 2 Diabetes Among Children and Adolescents From 2001 to 2009," *Journal of the American Medical Association*, 311, no. 17 (2014): 1778–86, DOI: 10.1001/jama.2014.3201.

70 S. Vijan et al., "Effect of Patients' Risks and Preferences on Health Gains with Glucose Lowering in Type 2 Diabetes," *JAMA Internal Medicine*, 174, no. 8 (2014): 1227–34, DOI: 10.1001/jamainternmed.2014.2894.

71   M. M. Poplawski et al., "Reversal of Diabetic Nephropathy by a Ketogenic Diet," *PLoS ONE*, 6, no. 4 (2011): e18604, DOI: 10.1371/journal.pone.0018604.

72   R. D. Feinman et al., "Dietary Carbohydrate Restriction as the First Approach in Diabetes Management: Critical Review and Evidence Base," *Nutrition*, 31, no. 1 (2015): 1–13, DOI: 10.1016/j.nut.2014.06.01.1.

73   "Making Healthy Food Choices: Grains and Starchy Vegetables," American Diabetes Association, http://www.diabetes.org/food-and-fitness/food/what-can-i-eat/making-healthy-food-choices/grains-and-starchy-vegetables.html, accessed November 28, 2016.

Appendix B

1   M. S. Touillaud et al., "Dietary Lignan Intake and Postmenopausal Breast Cancer Risk by Estrogen and Progesterone Receptor Status," *Journal of the National Cancer Institute*, 2007, 99(6):475–86, DOI: 10.1093/jnci/djk096.

2   A. Ahmad et al., "A Review on Therapeutic Potential of *Nigella Sativa:* A Miracle Herb," *Asian Pacific Journal of Tropical Biomedicine*, 2013, 3(5):337-352, DOI: .1016/S2221-1691(13)60075-1.

3   S. Hasani-Ranjbar, Z. Jouyandeh, and M. A. Abdollahi, "A Systematic Review of Anti-Obesity Medicinal Plants—An Update," *Journal of Diabetes and Metabolic Disorders*, 2013, 12:28, DOI: 10.1186/2251-6581-12-28.

4   M. Yadav et al., "Medicinal and biological Potential of Pumpkin: An Updated Review," *Nutrition Research Reviews*, 2010, 23(2), 184–90, DOI: 10.1017/S0954422410000107.

5   W. A. Morgan and B. J. Clayshulte, "Pecans Lower Low Density Lipoprotein Cholesterol in People with Normal Lipid Levels," *Journal of the American Dietetic Association*, March 2000, 100(3):312–18, DOI: 10.1016/S0002-8223(00)00097-3.

6   Oakridge Associated Universities, "Brazil Nuts," http://www.orau.org/PTP/collection/consumer%20products/brazilnuts.htm.

INDEX

ACKNOWLEDGMENTS

My intention for this book is to catalyze a revolution in how chronic diseases like cancer, heart and neurodegenerative diseases, diabetes, and obesity are treated.

Rather than rely on expensive symptomatic pharmacological approaches, I hope to empower patients and physicians with the practical tools to address mitochondrial dysfunction, the metabolic cause of most diseases.

I hope it will change the world by minimizing needless pain and suffering and helping restore mitochondrial function through metabolic optimization.

Although this book is not a scientific paper, I firmly believe in the benefit of peer review to confirm the accuracy of the information I'm presenting. Hence, I invited over 30 of the leading experts on this topic to review the text before it was submitted to the publisher. I am indebted to those who took the time to do so.

I have listed these cherished professionals below. They reviewed the text and provided many helpful suggestions that were integrated into the book.

Because the women and men listed below contributed so greatly to this book, I now publicly acknowledge their invaluable insights and assistance.

HEALTH PROFESSIONALS

Ron Rosedale, M.D.

Dr. Rosedale is founder of the Rosedale Center, co-founder of the Colorado Center for Metabolic Medicine (Boulder, CO) and founder of the Carolina Center of Metabolic Medicine (Asheville, NC). Through these centers, he has helped thousands suffering from so-called incurable diseases regain their health. He also created The Rosedale Diet, detailing the first "fasting mimetic" diet and his proven methods for treating diabetes, cardiovascular disease, arthritis, osteoporosis, and other chronic diseases of aging. One of Dr. Rosedale's life goals is to wipe out type 2 diabetes.

Dr. Rosedale was instrumental in helping me first understand the importance of insulin in 1995, and 20 years later the importance of limiting protein because of its impact on the mTOR signaling pathway.

Jason Fung, M.D.

Dr. Fung is a Toronto-based nephrologist. He completed medical school and internal medicine at the University of Toronto before finishing his nephrology fellowship at the University of California, Los Angeles at the Cedars-Sinai hospital. He joined Scarborough General Hospital in 2001, where he continues to practice. *The Complete Guide to Fasting*, of which he is the coauthor, is in my view the finest book written on the use of fasting in clinical practice. This is important, as fasting is one of the most profound interventions to jump-start your metabolism into burning fat as your primary fuel.

Robert Lustig, M.D, M.S.L.

Dr. Lustig is a professor of pediatrics in the division of endocrinology at the University of California, San Francisco, and former director of the Weight Assessment for Teen and Child Health (WATCH) Program at UCSF. He did a lecture in 2009 called

"Sugar: The Bitter Truth" that has been viewed 7 million times and brought great attention to the issue of excessive fructose as a metabolic toxin. He is also the author of *Fat Chance,* and his work on sugar has been covered on *60 Minutes.*

David Perlmutter, M.D.

Dr. Perlmutter is a board-certified neurologist and received his degree from the University of Miami School of Medicine. He is the recipient of the Linus Pauling award, and has authored four *New York Times* bestsellers including *Grain Brain: The Surprising Truth about Wheat, Carbs and Sugar,* with over 1 million copies in print. Others include *Brain Maker, The Grain Brain Cookbook,* and his most recent book, *The Grain Brain Whole Life Plan.*

Malcom Kendrick, M.D.

Dr. Kendrick, like me, is a family physician. He currently lives in Macclesfield, England, and has written two excellent books, *The Great Cholesterol Con* and *Doctoring Data.* He also blogs at drmalcolmkendrick.org where he explores a number of health issues, focusing primarily on cardiovascular disease.

Thomas Seyfried, Ph.D.

Dr. Seyfried is a professor of biology at Boston College and is a pioneer in the field of viewing cancer as a metabolic disease. He wrote the classic textbook on the topic, *Cancer as a Metabolic Disease.* It was a great privilege to have access to his expertise to untangle some of the complex science in this area.

Jeanne A. Drisko, M.D.

Dr. Drisko received her M.D. from the University of Kansas Medical Center, where she currently is the Rioridan Endowed Professor of Orthomolecular Medicine and Research and director of the KU Integrative Medicine Department since 1988.

William LaValley, M.D.

Dr. LaValley obtained his medical degree from Baylor College of Medicine in Houston, Texas, and is a licensed physician in Austin, Texas, and Nova Scotia, Canada, since 1988. He integrates evidence-based molecularly-targeted anti-cancer natural product supplements and repurposed anti-cancer pharmaceuticals for advanced molecular Integrative Oncology treatments in addition to (not instead of) conventional cancer care. Over the last 10 years Dr. LaValley has developed an extensive, state-of-the-art relational database that covers the molecular biology of cancer. He was instrumental in sending me the study that revealed the true mechanism of the action of insulin, which led to the development of the feast-famine cycle I described in Chapter 11.

Stephanie Seneff, Ph.D.

Dr. Seneff is a senior research scientist at the MIT Computer Science and Artificial Intelligence Laboratory and is an incredibly bright, innovative thinker who, among many other things, has done much work in describing how glyphosate, the active ingredient in the herbicide Roundup, causes harm in humans.

Miriam Kalamian, Ed.M., M.S., C.N.S.

Miriam is one of the leading nutritionists in the world in the practical application of nutritional ketosis for cancer. She has consulted with many hundreds of patients referred to her by Dr. Thomas Seyfried and Dr. Dominic D'Agostino, as well as a number of other prominent figures in the keto world, including low-carber Jimmy Moore. She is also creating a course to certify health professionals in nutritional ketosis through Certified Nutrition Specialists. I worked very closely with Miriam on most of the book to confirm its accuracy, and she was invaluable in the editing process.

Dan Pompa, D.C.

Dr. Pompa received his degree at Life University outside of Atlanta. He was an elite cyclist but developed chronic fatigue syndrome, which catalyzed his becoming an expert in cellular detoxification. He does not see patients but teaches hundreds of professionals how to implement this process that he integrates with nutritional ketosis. Because so many clinicians follow his protocols, he has one of the most extensive collections of information on the use of nutritional ketosis. While attending a conference in Orlando in September 2016, Dr. Pompa and I took a long walk and developed the feast-famine cycle component of the program I outline in this book. This portion of the program is largely based on his extensive clinical experience and is a key component of adopting the metabolic therapy over the long term.

Patricia Daly, m.B.A.N.T., r.C.H.N.C.

Patricia Daly is a cancer survivor and an experienced nutritional therapist specializing in the support of cancer patients and the ketogenic diet in particular. She has worked with hundreds of cancer patients in Ireland and abroad, lectures at the Irish Institute of Nutrition and Health, and is a well-regarded speaker at conferences and in cancer centers. *The Ketogenic Kitchen,* co-written with Domini Kemp, is her excellent book on practical suggestions for incorporating nutritional ketosis. Like Miriam, she has extensive experience in practical applications of nutritional ketosis.

Andrew Saul, Ph.D.

Dr. Saul has 40 years of experience in natural health education. He is the author of the popular books *Doctor Yourself* and *Fire Your Doctor* and coauthor of a dozen other books. His website, doctoryouself.com, is a comprehensive source of peer-reviewed natural health information. Dr. Saul is on the editorial board of the *Journal of Orthomolecular Medicine*, is editor-in-chief of the peer-reviewed Orthomolecular Medical News Service, and was elected in to the Orthomolecular Medicine Hall of Fame in 2013.

Michael Stroka, J.D., M.B.A., M.S., C.N.S., L.D.N.

Michael is an attorney, and is the only expert on this list who is a former patient of mine. After I helped him recover from a chronic debilitating illness, he shifted careers and is now the executive director of the Board for Certification of Nutrition Specialists, the organization that is providing the framework for the certification of professionals in the clinical use of nutritional ketosis.

Steve Haltiwanger, M.D., C.C.N.

Dr. Steven Haltiwanger is a physician and certified clinical nutritionist with over 25 years of practice. He is well known for his research on electrotherapy and is the health and science director of LifeWave. Dr. Haltiwanger has also extensively studied the effects of light therapy, magnetic field therapy and nutrient therapy on cell regeneration of biological tissue.

William Wilson, M.D.

Dr. Wilson is a family physician and graduate of the University of Minnesota medical school. He developed a disease model connecting food and brain function that he coins Carbohydrate Associated Reversible Brain syndrome, or CARB Syndrome. He is an active participant on my website and is passionate about the benefits of low-carb diets, so I invited him to review the manuscript.

OTHER PROFESSIONALS

Kate Hanley

Kate is an experienced health journalist and book collaborator, and was the primary editor of this book. I was most fortunate to have the opportunity to work with her, as she is beyond talented at converting complex medical topics into easy-to-understand text.

Barbara Loe Fisher

Barb is a treasured friend and champion of vaccine safety and the informed consent ethic. She is president of the National Vaccine Information Center (NVIC), a nonprofit charity she cofounded with parents of DPT vaccine injured children in 1982. She is one of the best editors I know, and her suggestions helped make the complex topics easier to digest.

Charlie Brown, J.D.

Charlie is another cherished friend who is the former attorney general of West Virginia and currently a tireless advocate for mercury-free dentistry. His organization, Consumers for Dental Choice, leads the campaign to abolish dental amalgam, a filling material that is 50 percent mercury. As president of the World Alliance for Mercury-Free Dentistry, he was instrumental in making sure the Minamata Convention on Mercury addressed amalgam. Like Barb, he is an excellent communicator and helped greatly with making the book easier to read.

Travis Christofferson

Travis is a gifted writer who wrote the book *Tripping over the Truth*, which played an important role in motivating me to write this book. I was familiar with most of the information he covered, but it never formed a cohesive narrative in my mind until I read his book. *Tripping over the Truth* is an important book to read for anyone who has cancer and is considering implementing metabolic therapy, as he provides the background information and framing perspective to help you understand the futility of the current cancer model, as well as the hope that metabolic therapy offers.

Aaron Davidson

Aaron is the programmer who created the Cronometer software that I feel is an essential tool for implementing the metabolic program that is outlined in the pages of this book. This free resource also helps collect data that will help me and other researchers further improve the approach.

ABOUT THE AUTHOR

Dr. Mercola is a true visionary who champions freedom of thought and of choice on all matters related to health. He has empowered millions of people around the world to take control of their health and has led the charge to implement much-needed changes to our current health-care system.

As a board-certified family physician for over three decades, Dr. Mercola treated many thousands of people at his wellness center where he focused on addressing the root cause of disease and encouraging patients to view food as medicine. In 1997, he founded his website, Mercola.com, which has become the most visited natural health website in the world and made him one the leading teachers of health. A three-time *New York Times* best-selling author, Dr. Mercola has appeared on CNN, Fox News, ABC News, *Today*, CBS's *Washington Unplugged*, and *The Dr. Oz Show*.

Hay House Titles of Related Interest

YOU CAN HEAL YOUR LIFE, the movie, starring Louise Hay & Friends
(available as a 1-DVD program, an expanded 2-DVD set,
and an online streaming video)
Learn more at www.hayhouse.com/louise-movie

THE SHIFT, the movie, starring Dr. Wayne W. Dyer
available as a 1-DVD program, an expanded 2-DVD set,
and an online streaming video)
Learn more at www.hayhouse.com/the-shift-movie

♦ ♦

*THE ALLERGY SOLUTION: Unlock the Surprising Hidden Truth
about Why You Are Sick and How to Get Well,*
by Leo Galland, M.D., and Jonathan Galland, J.D.

*GODDESSES NEVER AGE: The Secret Prescription for Radiance,
Vitality, and Well-Being,* by Christiane Northrup, M.D.

*THE REAL FOOD REVOLUTION: Healthy Eating,
Green Groceries, and the Return of the American Family Farm,*
by Congressman Tim Ryan

*YOUNG AND SLIM FOR LIFE: 10 Essential Steps to Achieve Total
Vitality and Kick-Start Weight Loss That Lasts,* by Frank Lipman, M.D.

All of the above are available at your local bookstore,
or may be ordered by contacting Hay House (see next page).

♦ ♦

We hope you enjoyed this Hay House book. If you'd like to receive our online catalog featuring additional information on Hay House books and products, or if you'd like to find out more about the Hay Foundation, please contact:

Hay House, Inc., P.O. Box 5100, Carlsbad, CA 92018-5100
(760) 431-7695 or (800) 654-5126
(760) 431-6948 (fax) or (800) 650-5115 (fax)
www.hayhouse.com® • www.hayfoundation.org

———

Published in Australia by:
Hay House Australia Pty. Ltd., 18/36 Ralph St., Alexandria NSW 2015
Phone: 612-9669-4299 • *Fax:* 612-9669-4144 • www.hayhouse.com.au

Published in the United Kingdom by:
Hay House UK, Ltd., Astley House, 33 Notting Hill Gate, London W11 3JQ
Phone: 44-20-3675-2450 • *Fax:* 44-20-3675-2451 • www.hayhouse.co.uk

Published in India by: Hay House Publishers India,
Muskaan Complex, Plot No. 3, B-2, Vasant Kunj, New Delhi 110 070
Phone: 91-11-4176-1620 • *Fax:* 91-11-4176-1630 • www.hayhouse.co.in

———

Access New Knowledge.
Anytime. Anywhere.

Learn and evolve at your own pace
with the world's leading experts.

www.hayhouseU.com

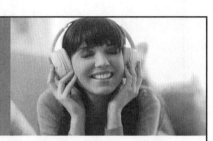

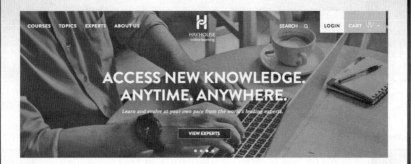
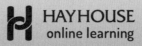